The Bird's Road

Sharek Amalek Gadd

Published by Inkshares, Inc., Oakland, California
www.inkshares.com

Edited by RaAnn Gadd, Morgan Ra Meredith, Elizabeth Judd,
Barbara Schirmer, and Nicole Hildreth
Cover design by Sharek A. Gadd
Author photo credit: Michael Durr / michaeldurr.com
Interior design by Kevin G. Summers

ISBN: 9781950301355
e-ISBN: 9781950301362
LCCN: 2021938944

First edition

Printed in the United States of America

To the long line of durable souls who passed the torch, generation after generation, and those who may rise when I fall:

There is no requirement to circumnavigate the globe to save humankind or sacrifice all that you are to benefit the world; all you have to do to pluck someone from damnation is to be welcoming. Be amenable to letting a child follow you around, sit on your porch, and hug your dog. Understand that little ones are more gifted than they could ever imagine and permit them to put their hands to some work. Fill that hole in your heart by sharing the things that make you shine; there's always someone out there who needs some light. Investigate the faces that life disfigured; there's an avenue of healing in that gaze. Call on the infirm and help them sift through their station. Be a friend to those outside your bonds, and don't be afraid of being injured or demeaned. Consider where you stand and realize you aren't the only traveler. Be aware that the individual who wants to control another person is struggling to manage their own. When you fail to navigate an obstacle, there's invariably someone nearby who knows the path. Never offer pity but be willing to share the burden. Don't be afraid to ask direct questions but be ready to welcome what's spoken. Know that the only heaven or hell to experience is on this earth and that the mirrors you pass reflect the only savior or devil there is. Reach beyond your grasp; you'll receive a library to learn in the falling.

CONTENTS

PROLOGUE

August 11, 2020

UNTIL NOW, I'VE never shared my whole story. For more than half my life, I didn't want anyone knowing anything about me.

There are occasions when people question my past, but I must temper what or how much I tell them. I've learned that bringing my experiences into a conversation affects it negatively. It's like pulling the pin from a grenade and setting it between us; after the blast, the recipients are generally left in disbelief or stammering with shock, not knowing what to say. To repair the awkward situation I create, I'm sure to patch them up by telling them I'm doing fine. In the end, I wish I had never had the exchange; the action takes more than it ever gives.

Sometimes they ask, "How did you survive?" or state, "I could never go through that."

Honestly, I don't know why I'm here. I didn't consciously do anything to stay alive. I'm even responsible for a few actions that lessened my chances of being here or peeled off years from the end of my life. I know I did more wrong than I ever did right, but here I am.

As a boy, I didn't understand the developments happening around me, and as a teen, I tried to ignore predicaments or, like pulling your hand away from a hot surface, intentionally forget them as soon as they occurred. How could I have known the recipe for survival that my childhood mind concocted could be so self-destructive? By the time I was a young man, these unaddressed accumulating injuries hobbled me like a prisoner in shackles.

Looking back, a lot of it seems trivial, but then, it wasn't, it was mountainous. Besides my immature qualities, there were several factors working against me. There were several factors working against all of us.

I understand many misfortunes happen without reason—that's a reality as far back as you can imagine and as far forward as you can't—but I've endured a lot of unreasonable things at such a pace or frequency that they seem natural to me. Truthfully, accounting for the changes they produced in me, and recognizing how they altered my outlook and patterned my decision-making process, cause much regret. Out of deep-rooted fear and anger, I chose to do a few things and to not do a lot of things. More often than not, I've gotten out of the boat when I should have sailed. I consistently went in one direction where a sensible person tacked the other way. I ran when I should have walked. I've taken when I should have given, and I've given things I should have kept.

What started as a simple recording of my history turned into a reckoning with my past. To come to terms with what twisted me, I needed to make space to investigate my path. After all, how can you ever know where you're going if you don't know where you've been? Time and distance enabled me to bear the weight, but I'd be lying if I didn't admit unpackaging this material hurt and brought tears while writing about things that happened forty years ago. Many times, I've asked myself, "Why do this—why plunge my hand to the bottom of the pool and stir the muck?" At times it's felt like an interrogation, if not torture. I've spent countless predawn hours following trails to subjects I never wanted to weep over or witness. A lot of my memories are difficult to access; imagine needing to swim submerged in a flooded cave, forcing your chest into a crack with no room to move your arms or turn around, trying to find a way through, but there's no light, and the only air is the last breath you took. It's a self-punishing challenge to recover heartbreaking parcels I sank as a boy.

When my life finally found structure on the screen of my secondhand laptop, I felt real. I felt like I did exist. I could see my childhood self, rooting around trying to find a way to be alive, but more than that, I could see all the souls around me struggling to do the same. I realized I shouldn't satisfy myself with merely seeing my story; I wanted to share theirs and what it was like to go with them where we went.

Even though I feel driven to publish these pages, I still hold a considerable amount of trepidation about you reading them. There's much in here that is my inner voice; at times, it's angry, often malicious, and sounds incredibly hurtful, but everything it spoke against felt the same. I'm accustomed to carrying everything that happened within myself, but having come this far, there's no sense in hiding it anymore. I know it's time to let it go.

I'm one of two remaining reliquaries of a family that no longer exists; within thirty years, most of the firsthand accounts of their moments on this earth will cease. Without these passages, no one will ever know their joys, struggles, or desires. They were amazing, in the greatest and simplest ways. Their hearts pounded, they cried, acted wildly, loved, made mistakes, hurt and tried to heal each other, bore children, and warred against circumstances they had no chance of defeating.

Writing this was a substantial challenge, especially for a nonwriter. There are lots of starts and stops, dates, ages, strange names, switches in time, and confusing subject matter—some of it's difficult for me to grasp, and some memories are still missing. To anticipate questions you may have later, I begin with a history (Chapter 1) handed to me from my Mom and Dad; it's a compilation from conversations, notebooks, journals, and handwritten entries on the backsides of tattered photographs. It reads as fragmented, but I didn't want to take away or add anything. Those passages are their stories, but they helped shape what I am. Everything after the first chapter is my perspective; you'll have your own, but be aware that what you're about to read is the internal conflict of a simple mind in the middle of a storm.

Thank you for picking up this book and making your way this far. Possibly by reading to the end, you'll encounter some small point that can shine a light in your darkness and help you navigate a path. There are characters here who did what they did, with what they had, under the burdens only they could carry. Perhaps, down your road, you'll think about the people I've known, how they engaged with the world, how they treated one another, and how they affected me. Maybe if you remember them, they'll have an opportunity to live well beyond their short lives.

Here is my story.

INTRODUCTION

1976 (Five Years Old)

WE WERE OUT of the house before dawn. The grass, wet with dew, was cold on my bare feet. I felt the mush of worm dirt on my soles. The breath of night air hung heavy, and it was quiet except for the crickets in the weeds. Dad's hand enveloped mine as I leaned my head against his hip. He wanted to show me something in the sky. We moved through the trees to find an unobstructed view. He pointed to the eastern horizon and described a collection of stars. I had a hard time discerning what he wanted me to see, but I listened to his description.

He said, "Orion is rising, and he's carrying the Bird's Road on his shoulder."

He crouched beside me, placed his forearm against the side of my head, and told me to look along its length to where his finger extended. It took a minute, but the constellation finally revealed itself. Off its right shoulder, I saw a glowing light that arced across the diamond-studded blackness.

Dad said, "What looks like a cloud over Orion's shoulder is the Bird's Road. Some people say the birds use it to travel by night. Some people used to believe it's where the soul flies when they die. I think we'll all go there at some point. That's where everything came from, and eventually it'll all find its way back."

I was five years old when he introduced me to the aggregation of starlight cast through our galactic plane. That type of impromptu education came readily from my dad. As a boy, I didn't understand most of his teaching—his words were cryptic and laced with spiritual references—and by the time I was a teen, his training made me shrink away. He had a way of using the minimum number of words at a critical point in time to peel away my clouded thoughts and sink a jewel of wisdom into my mind. Most of these instances revolved around some trauma, as if the event held a spike for him to drive home. His lessons often hurt me, but the same way a tree must feel when it's pruned after a storm or a fowl when it's forced to molt by the change of seasons. He could counsel tenderly, but those moments were rare.

He carefully considered everything around him and enjoyed sharing his opinions. Most of his thoughts were common, but some he held close as they were too deep to fathom or were on the fringe of reason. One of those guarded suspicions was that we are all fragments of the same stone or like embers kicked from some fire at the dawn of creation. Another of his ruminations was that we'd all lived previous lives, connected by genetic memory. He dabbled in numerology and past-life regression but rooted himself with a sound and intelligent mind.

He often talked about a person's fiber and believed an individual's character wasn't original but was like a patchwork quilt, made from a multitude of experiences. He spoke of how to be a human being and the cost of living forever; he reflected on those sentiments and affirmed that the only acceptable currency is influence. You've got to mean something to people.

Good or bad, when you affect someone, you'll always reside somewhere in their mind. If you're hurtful to them, they'll curse your eternity—be their friend in the darkness, and you'll shimmer with the angels. If you're willing to walk either of those roads, a stranger's offspring will speak of you and share your story, generation after generation.

Dad would say, "If you want to understand a person, and most certainly yourself, you have to look at all the insignificant things that one's keen to hold or do—there's reason in the unreasonable. People and their stories are important; pay attention to them and don't be quick to judge. They may have had a rough upbringing or suffered at the hands of others—maybe they've lived like a dream and have the ability to heal the world of its wounds. They will, most likely, have something to teach you. If you look closely enough and think deeply enough, you'll most likely learn it. You'll be bettered by it."

I didn't need much encouragement to observe or listen. Everything was fascinating, be it light moving through a room, a dog on a trail, or how a person's nose moved when they told a story. I enjoyed the voices around me and the way they spoke. I loved people that others liked, and the unloved bewitched me. I paid thought to the little things people mentioned in passing; like a thief, I collected their interests as my own.

Maybe he was thinking about my sisters that morning. Perhaps he was thinking about his mom and dad, or what he'd lost as a boy. Maybe he was giving me a way to remember something important. I don't believe he had any premonitions, but it was evident he felt something moving within our family, and it was as beautiful as it was horrific. It was as brilliant and as dark as the sky that night.

CHAPTER 1

Foundations
1906–1973

MY FATHER'S MOTHER, Stella De Luz, was a Portuguese immigrant. She was slight, not much more than five feet tall, with raven hair and skin the color of tobacco. She was five years old, in 1906, when she and her family boarded a tall ship and sailed from the Azores to resettle in the Territory of Hawaii. By the time the westerly winds rolled the wooden vessel on its side while rounding Cape Horn, the seas were as black as the faces on the bodies stored in the hold for burial on reaching their destination.

Stella's family, indentured by the Hawaiian Sugar Planters' Association, agreed to exchange labor in the Oahu sugarcane fields for the cost of their passage and room and board during their tenure. With thousands of others, they lived in little shacks propped up on stilts to keep them cool and the vermin from easily entering. The endeavor required all able bodies—even children—to participate. She and her siblings received half the credit of an adult by sewing sacks or killing rats that infested the cane expanses. The bookmen logged the credits at the company store where workers could swap them for food, sundries, and rent, but they never earned enough to pay off their initial debts. Stella was fortunate; her plantation provided education. Between plantings and harvests, she learned a trade, working as a dental technician in the camp infirmary. She was fifteen when she met her beau, Charles Gadd, a rawboned and lanky Kentuckian.

As a soldier, Charles survived France during the Great War and the influenza pandemic of 1918. The Army stationed him at Fort Shafter, the first military garrison on Oahu. Known as a ladies' man, he collected flowers from several girls in the tropical paradise and pursued Stella. They courted for a significant part of his tour and married in 1923.

They wore floral leis on the day they departed the island chain. A steamship bore them to San Francisco, and a coal-fired train delivered them to Charles's hometown of Berea, Kentucky. They moved into a board-and-batten shack on the neglected end of town, where Charles turned to the business of cutting timber and siring offspring.

The hardships of the 1930s challenged Charles and ended his vocation in the lumber industry. This pinched his scant resources, and his children felt the pangs of cold and hunger. When the logging companies migrated north, he uprooted his family and followed the promise of gainful employment to Martinsville, Indiana. The mill offered them a home on the south side of the rail tracks in an area called Bucktown.

Although the scenery changed, the struggle was the same, and Charles's vice of alcohol did little to settle the troubles ruling his mind. Some people said it was the war that reforged Charles and gave him a soldier's heart, and maybe it did, but it was no excuse for his actions. He was callous, if not cruel, and his hands channeled frustration on his weary wife and seven children.

#

Stella gave birth to my father, George Charles, on October 1, 1939. He took after Stella, being short, slim, and dark-skinned. As he grew, she and George developed a sweet relationship. He liked to help her; he gathered water in pails to keep in the kitchen and split kindling for the stove. In the winter, he broke the ice in the well barrel and swept out the snow that drifted in under the doors.

Food was scarce, and they made ends meet by eating things most people gave to their hogs; weeds, turkey necks, chicken feet, gizzards, and squirrels—recovered from the house cat's clutches—staved off hunger.

In the spring of 1950, Stella's performance during her chores slowed, and she lost more weight than a lack of nourishment could explain. George thought she was hungry, and Charles believed she was lazy. At night, from the bed he shared with his brother, George helplessly listened as his father viciously abused his mother. Two years later, a doctor diagnosed Stella with cancer. She may have been hungry, but she wasn't lazy. She quickly declined. George was twelve when Stella died.

Charles, always a scoundrel, kept several ladies around town. Days after Stella's passing, he figured it best to send his children away to make space for a paramour and her gaggle of kids.

George, now homeless, found ways to shelter and feed himself; he visited local churches on Sundays for an occasional meal, introduced himself to old-timers that paid him to wrangle repairs on their homes, and delivered groceries for the neighborhood store. He stayed on his feet while daylight persisted, kept up his appearance by utilizing the gymnasium showers, and when he couldn't stay awake any longer, he'd find a shed or barn where he could sneak a few hours of sleep. When winter came, he had nowhere to go but to his brother, Amos. Amos's wife traded George a room for the greater portion of his income but locked him from the residence while she and Amos partied on the weekends. While wandering the streets, three frozen nights out of each week, he hatched a plan to hide part of his weekly wages in a tobacco tin to buy himself a house. Eventually, with his hidden savings, George purchased a crippled car that served him as a home. He lived in his sedan and continued scraping by with odd jobs and the generosity of friends. George maintained his schoolwork and was a fixture in the town that people expected to see. When he was out of sight, there was concern for his welfare.

#

My maternal grandparents, Carl and Garnet Stanger, came from German stock. Both were tall, broad-shouldered, and adorned with dazzling blue eyes and exceptional features. Carl was twice a veteran. Under the minimum age and using an assumed name, he enlisted in the Army. He labored in the Panama Canal Zone but while home on furlough, he refused to return to his company and they declared him absent without leave (AWOL). The guns of the First World War called Carl back to arms through a legitimate enlistment, where he served in France as a wagoner. Being honorably discharged after the war, he returned to Paragon, Indiana, and promptly married a fifteen-year-old, Dozy Garnet Lietzman. Garnet hailed from a family of farmers that embraced fidelity and inclined toward hard toil.

My grandparents lived on the same end of town as George's father, but their home was more refined than the neighboring structures. Its exterior, clad in clapboard siding, held the weather at bay. The plastered interior, warmed not only by a coal stove but also by several industrious children, was comfortable.

#

My mother, Jerra—twelve years younger than her nearest sibling—was more like a daughter to some of them, and they treated her like one. She met my father when she was twelve and he was fourteen. They were fast friends and soon more than fond of being together.

During the winter of George's third high school year, he contracted pneumonia and lay dying out of view. Jerra, concerned by his absence, tasked her brother Carl with her fears. He found George, near death, within the frosted confines of his car. Garnet and Carl brought George to their home to recuperate and, from that point forward, knitted him into the Stanger family.

George's qualities endeared him as another son to Carl and Garnet, and he whiled away his hours within his newfound family. Hunting and sporting with Carl and experiencing the care and concern from a would-be mother filled a grievous absence in my father's heart.

#

George received his diploma, took a job as an apprentice machinist, and enrolled in trade school. Even though he was fully invested in earning a wage, the center of his world was Jerra. They married when he was eighteen and she was sixteen and moved to Indianapolis to be closer to George's work and study. Their first child was my sister, Carrie. She arrived on July

30, 1959. Carrie, like our mother, was blue eyed with golden curls. She was cheerful and tumbled happily along with my parents and their rapid succession of life events.

Not quite a year after Carrie came into the world, my sister Garnna was born. Her eyes and hair were dark, like our father's. Thirteen months after Garnna's birth, right about the time she took her first steps and sweetly chattered as babies do, a seemingly ordinary fever troubled her. My parents figured it was from teething but tried to keep Garnna's head and neck cool. Within twenty-four hours, her blood roiled and turned her olive complexion to fire while she screamed and vomited. The next morning, while my father was at work, waves of convulsions racked Garnna. My mother and a neighbor rushed her to Riley Children's Hospital; when they arrived, she was limp and unconscious.

Within hours of admitting her for care, the attending physician determined that Garnna was in an outmatched fight with spinal meningitis. Half a day later, the medical staff informed my father they held no hope for her recovery. He was twenty-one when he removed Garnna from life support. Weeping bitterly, he poured tears over the daughter that was so full of joy just a few days before. He cradled her in his arms and caressed her brow as her spirit departed like water through a sieve.

My mother was nineteen on a bright August day when she watched Garnna's little body lowered into the ground. For months, nightmares of Garnna buried alive haunted Jerra. Garnna's daily absence troubled her three-year-old sister; Carrie cried for her missing playmate. The last time Carrie questioned the lack of her sister's presence, she and my mother were folding Garnna's remaining articles and placing them into the bottom of a drawer. At that point, Carrie seemed to understand that her sister wasn't coming home.

#

As the days accumulated behind my parents, the addition of children rounded the sharp pains of loss. Jerra was pregnant when Garnna died. Her first son, Daniel Charles, was born on the twenty-fourth of June 1962, and the following year, Jerra delivered Joseph Michael on the twenty-fifth of September 1963. Danny looked like a miniature George, and Joe took after our mother. Four-year-old Carrie was her father's daughter and knitted to him whenever he was home. The boys combined forces and were a whirlwind of mischief, scattering toddler-sized damage wherever they ventured. They were content and lived as peacefully as a young family is able, in a factory house on the west end of Indianapolis.

#

At three years of age, Joe's stature increased abnormally. He quickly outpaced Danny in size and strength and exhibited signs of puberty. With great concern, my parents pressed Joe's pediatrician for answers. After almost a year of tests and studies, the doctor offered that Joe showed symptoms of gigantism and chanced to think there was an issue with Joe's pituitary gland. He scheduled exploratory surgery at Riley Hospital, where the surgical team found and removed a tumor. The clinic determined the tumor was benign and suggested monthly visits to monitor Joe's health. The procedure remedied Joe's abnormal growth, but not his penchant for being overly helpful and sneaking out of the house in his Halloween costume to collect candy from neighbors. Danny eventually grew to match Joe's size, and life went on without extraordinary challenges.

Spiritualism

My father was a spiritual man and involved in Christianity since he was a teen. The religion, wrought from arduous experiences, and structured not to take lightly, shaped his mind. Forgiveness of transgressions wasn't by grace, and only those that sacrificed convenience and modern pleasures reserved their place in heaven. The path to the hereafter, like a tightrope over a void, challenged the average person. The slovenly were seldom able to cross the chasm, which is this life on earth.

His mother was a Catholic, but George was never christened in that church. Searching for security in his life while living alone, he stumbled into the local Pentecostal church and adopted their ways. He met my mother in that building and worshipped there until my grandfather, Carl, was embroiled in a doctrinal disagreement with the presiding pastor. My father solved Carl's quandary by transporting him to another parish in town, a communal sect, led by the "movement of the Spirit."

David Warrant was the pastor of this new congregation, and he had the kind of charisma that drew men and women to him like moths to a flame. David was soft-spoken and intelligent. He could turn almost anyone to his way. Some held him as a prophet of old or as one touched by God. David was a reader of the human condition and was also a student of psychology and political philosophy. He understood the vices that debased people and the ideals that elevated them. He also realized the weakness, pain, and desperation that caused individuals to reach beyond their grasp, and he placed himself in the gap to offer God's Divine Assistance.

#

David's Martinsville church meetings were a satellite venture of the larger organization he shepherded in Indianapolis. His Indianapolis church building was on the same block as the People's Temple, pastored by the infamous Reverend James Warren Jones. Jim Jones and David were contemporaries but of different cloth, though both moved their supple flocks toward coarse pastures.

Young and vibrant, the religious subculture of the era wanted spiritual and community solutions to bring them out of tired Christian dogma. They also sought to free themselves from the damage of waning morals, the Vietnam War, and societal decay. They gave themselves a considerable challenge and hoped for a libertarian's reward.

In the late 1960s, Jim and David peppered their sermons with comparisons of modern societies' trappings and values to "skag" (heroin) and its addictive qualities. They drew the correlation that, if you're in this world, you're hooked on skag, and becoming free meant you must withdraw. Feverish admonitions to further separate themselves from skag came readily.

Reverend Jones and David were familiar with the ideals of Apostolic Communalism; again, the social terrain was fertile for utopian dreams to take hold. Jones moved his charge to California and on to horrific infamy, while David's flock—swindled by an unscrupulous landlord—vacated Indianapolis.

#

David had found a place for his church to gather in Wilbur, Indiana. While the congregation refurbished the buildings in Wilbur, David was "Led by the Spirit" and discovered an overgrown homestead nestled in the forests of southern Indiana. It contained eighty-six acres, a rough-hewn barn, and a derelict, ninety-year-old farmhouse.

On entering the site, David's God spoke to him, saying, "In this place, men will take off their shoes."

David accepted this as a call to action and returned to his congregation with plans to acquire the found property as soon as possible.

#

My mother and father maintained their relationship with David's church and invested in spirituality, family, and community ideals. When the congregation moved to Wilbur, my parents commuted to the small hamlet.

During this period, my father received a troubling vision. The dream wouldn't leave him when he woke and stayed with him for years afterward. The subconscious display wasn't the simple rehash of emotions concerning daily events and easily interpreted actions; a voice spoke to him in the dream, and the clarity of the imagery and the intensity of the feelings were vexing.

My father described the event: "I was standing in a great fog of fear and dread. I looked into the horror where, out of the mist, the shape of a boy took form, and I heard a voice speak, 'Lamech.' Shortly thereafter, a second boy emerged from the gloom, and the voice spoke again, 'Amalek.' Eventually, the two boys faded into the darkness, and I awoke with a shudder."

My father carried this dream, failing to understand its meaning, but recognized that it was significant. On the seventh of January 1967, when Jerra birthed their next (fifth) child, a son, George named the boy Lamech.

Padanaram

The property David and his followers purchased in 1966, he named Padanaram. In the Old Testament, Padanaram (the Plain of Aram) was a geographic region where Abraham and his progeny obtained their wives. Though it was assigned a biblical label, they commonly called the commune "The Valley."

An avian view of the Valley would lead you to believe its terrain is of the average Indiana fare, but if you walked there, you would attest that it owns a unique quality. It exudes an energy that calls to recollection legends of creation. The contours of the scenery are a sacred geometry that always gives you the perfect vantage. The landscape nurses genetic memories that whisper to your soul in a forgotten language.

Its forest covers the foundation of an ancient seabed. For unfathomable years, torrents of glacial melt and rain cleaved and washed the ground, forming channels and coves. The waters exposed aquifers and secreted caves from which sweet springs tumble. Mosses and ferns blanket the worn stone and retain ages of rich loam.

Sulfur Creek, as they call it now, is a weak remnant of the icy inundation that sculpted the place. The creek's course slinks lazily through the Valley's plain, meandering back on itself, over and over, like a giant serpent resting in the sun. Small green fish dart above the sandy bed of the sun-dappled brook as if defending the cool abode from prying eyes. Crawfish tend their gardens under equisetum (horsetail) banks, while dragonflies and swallows skip and dive along the shimmering surface. Copperheads and water snakes insinuate up the smaller spring branches, angling for minnows and frogs.

Eons ago, megafauna migrated through the valley, followed by bands of skin-clad humans. The migratory hunters camped and tracked their prey from under fire-lit rock shelters, leaving their detritus as path markers for succeeding generations.

Migrants from another continent who hacked their way from the east succeeded those first nomads, following the old trails into the Valley. They built a hewn cabin and a large barn from poplar and beech, drank from the springs, and tilled the grass-covered flats with oxen. A cholera epidemic soon silenced their sounds of toil. The only witnesses to their passage were the creek swaying through its course, whip-poor-wills calling in the night, crickets and cicadas sighing, and the wind rattling the grasses.

The pioneers' rectangular structures, being disassembled by insects, vines, and weather, remained for another age until David found them. As new settlers, David's followers personalized the process of taking dominion over the Valley. They hunted, planted crops, and established the ideals that kept order in the settlement. They sold what possessions they held and offered the funds for distribution as David saw fit. They renovated the ancillary buildings and filled the barn with cattle and hogs.

Communism

My father completed his education and was a journeyman in the tool and die trades. My mother delivered a fifth child, Lamech, and was already pregnant with her sixth baby. They spent their free time in Padanaram and wanted to grow with the venture, so they forfeited their possessions, cast their lot with David, and rooted themselves in the commune.

When they settled there, it was a challenging existence; there were food and shelter but still a need for human-made sundries, such as cloth, hardware, healthcare items, and fuel. The community hatched a plan to peddle natural resources the Valley offered. They could sell unrefined wood to local mills for quick cash, so they set about clearing the terrain. The focus of the inhabitants turned from spiritualism to selling timber.

My father engineered and built a ripsaw from stonecutting equipment salvaged from a defunct stone quarry in the nearby town of Bedford. They planted this machinery in the center of the Valley, and it became the heart of the colony. The mill roared from first light into the dark of night.

Testimony of the commune spread, and people from all corners of the country came to live in its confines. Medical students, nurses, teachers, mechanics, and electricians made their way to the Valley and provided critical services. Some of these wanderers assimilated, but most failed to maintain their existence as the daily toil was harsh. Duties were assigned along gender lines; the males wrangled the property's business and harvested livestock and wild game, while the females maintained the domiciles and burdened themselves with the inhabitants' tutelage and feeding. My father worked as a labor foreman. He was an honest taskmaster, but many of the recent arrivals misjudged him as a tyrant. He held close to one of the establishment's central tenets: *If you don't work, you will not eat.* If an individual wasn't at their designated location by their scheduled hour, he'd find them and if need be, drag them to their station.

When the commune became self-sufficient, they wrought together massive log buildings and planted them in the fertile ground. Like organic stave churches, multistoried dormitories for unmarried men and women rose to the sky. Diminutive two-story family structures peppered the settlement, and the appearance of the area was that of an Old Norse village.

#

On the twenty-second of October 1970, my father delivered his sixth child, Shelam, with a midwife's oversight. She carried the character and image of her father with her demeanor and dark complexion. She was cheerful, chubby, and talkative. Shelam sang songs and engaged in conversations with Lamech's pet mynah bird. She became the warmth and light inside our poplar cabin. If joy were a physical quantity, she was every bit its match. She ensnared us with her spirit.

#

These days were enjoyable, but the pleasure was fleeting. With the influx of people at Padanaram, the work burden wasn't as heavy, but a cultural change was underway. In 1970, the new arrivals included characters possessing weak ethics and an inclination to abuse drugs. My father had his hands full with the upkeep of the mill machinery and the forest operations. Added to his responsibilities were teams of new arrivals that bucked at his leadership. My mother managed the care and rearing of five children and her everyday duties concerning the commune's welfare, and, once more, she was pregnant.

Shelam

In February 1971, my brother Joe was due for an appointment with his pediatrician, and the laundry dryers in the commune were down for repairs. My mother—four months into her seventh pregnancy—planned a consolidated trip to address both issues. She bundled Shelam for the weather, noticing her hat was too tight to fit, as Joe loaded wet clothes into the car.

With Joe's eighth-year evaluation completed, they walked next door to the laundromat. My mother dried and folded clothing while Joe played with Shelam on the tile floor. The task was warm and peaceful until Joe screamed for Mom's attention. Mom rounded the corner of the sorting table and found fourteen-month-old Shelam cramped in a grand mal seizure. Horrified with flashbacks of Garnna, my mother scooped her from the ground and, with Joe, rushed back to the pediatrician's office.

An X-ray depicted an enormous tumor in the rear of Shelam's brain. She required emergency surgery, and they immediately transferred her to Riley Children's Hospital in Indianapolis. After the operation, the surgeon informed my parents he couldn't remove the entire mass, and the biopsy confirmed that it was malignant. He explained, with great sadness, there was nothing more he could do for Shelam but comfort her pain. They expected the rapidly expanding cancer to consume her within six months.

For weeks, Shelam remained unconscious and was unresponsive as my parents held vigil at the hospital. Eventually, she moved her hands—searching across the sheets—and finally called for her blanket. Her eyes were unfocused but tracked sound through the room. That's when they found that the surgery's invasiveness had destroyed her vision and left her blind. After caring for Shelam for more than a month, the hospital staff relented to my parents' pleas that they be allowed to carry Shelam home to die.

#

Wildflowers erupting from the forest loam and robins heralding their return offered hope after a frigid winter. The sun cast its light on the Valley floor and caressed the emergent life but did little to warm our hearts. Shelam was home but not expected to live to the autumn. Mostly, she was unaffected by her blindness but suffered discomfort, noticeable on her furrowed brow.

When the pain made her irritable and inconsolable, my mother treated her with Demerol.

We felt isolated and hopeless inside our hovel, and people outside the cabin compounded the situation. The appearance of death in a child tested many that professed love of all creation, including the ill and infirm; they withered under its power. Hushed conversations and outright protestations made it known Shelam wasn't welcome in the dining hall and communal areas.

#

My mother was eight months into her last pregnancy when she fell and fractured her leg while carrying Shelam on a dew-covered path. This injury confined her to the cabin during the sweltering month of June, until my birth on July 1, 1971. After my delivery, a surgeon in Bedford relieved her of her cast and set her ankle with pins. A week in the hospital gave her respite from the conditions at home.

Although uncomfortable, August was sweet. Shelam regained the ability to sit upright and was jovial. She learned her world through touch and sound and could recognize our noises and called to us. She was excited by the new baby she could hear beside her. Lamech spent most of his time reading books to Shelam and was her constant companion. She adored him.

#

The changing light and air of September brought with it a coolness that also settled upon Shelam. She slept throughout the day and refused to eat.

By October, Shelam was wasting away. Swelling disfigured her head, and she was listless. Her magpie voice never offered sound again.

#

My mother fell into a dark depression. Prostrated by injury and grief, she lay between Shelam and her new child. The profound reality of being anchored between life and death broke her spirit. Like a dog barking in the night, she called to a god that ignored her pleas. Garnna's end, some years before, was like a flash of lighting that gave no warning, and its lack of anticipation left her with only the challenge of recovery. Shelam's situation was far more crushing; each day wore on by minutes, and the sorrow and hurt came like waves to a castaway mariner on an unending ocean.

#

Seeds of anger and disgust toward David and Padanaram's workings found purchase in my parents' hearts. The revenue that the logging and lumber operations procured went into the commune infrastructure, and David distributed the remainder among the members to buy necessities. My family's disbursement wasn't enough to cover Shelam's expenses, so my father went to David with the issue. David refused to pay the doctors and the hospital that treated Shelam. David called it "robbing skag" (permissibly stealing from the world), but to my father, that was ignorance and an insult to the people that tried to save Shelam. Her care was paramount, and the relationships with the physicians needed fostering. Failure to render payment was not an option, and Dad now knew his labor at the sawmill was unfruitful. He maintained his shifts cutting timber but hired on to a machine shop in Bedford and worked a night shift to settle his bills. He also took upon himself feeding Shelam through a tube. From this point forward, this was how she received nutrients and medication. Once again, Dad cradled a dying child.

#

The leaves fell in November, and December brought freezing rain and cold. The woods were barren, and Shelam's breathing turned shallow and slow. January was white and bitter. The chill outside seemed to creep inside the dark walls and permeate our souls. Shelam's departure felt close. The doctor didn't understand how she remained alive, and we didn't either. The pediatrician supposed that the only thing keeping her tied to this world was the love showered on her. Her connection to life was like a single strand of filament spun by a spider. This mooring was so succinct that movement and words became hushed as if a mere vibration would break the thread.

#

Shelam's state was tenuous but had become routine. Our condition extracted an emotional toll on my mother, and now it imposed a physical tax; her nails fell from her fingers.

On the twenty-fifth of January 1971, my mother departed the Valley for Bedford to see a practitioner about her hands. While in town, freezing rain fell. By the time she left the doctor's office and made her way to State Road 58, ice had formed a thick sheet on the winding trace, completely covering the fifteen miles to the commune.

State Road 58 was originally a wagon trail, hacked out of the forest by settlers; it's full of switchbacks and off-camber turns. The course is a twenty-minute jaunt in pleasant conditions, but inclement weather can quickly turn the path into an arduous, hours-long expedition.

My mother inched along, looking for traction. The route was vacant except for a black vehicle in the distance. The driver of the vehicle was evidently unfamiliar with the passage, and my mother eventually gained on their position. On a curve in the road through the trees, she spied the automobile and realized she was following a coroner's hearse. Sorrow poured from her when she understood that there was only one place the hearse could be going. She crumpled in agony, and tears wet her face as she followed the coal-colored wagon, mile by crushing mile, to Padanaram's lane and our cabin door.

The faint sinew holding Shelam to this world unraveled in the absence of my mother. We wept as the undertaker lay Shelam in the hearse's chamber. The months of worry and battered emotions found an end. Shelam, our chubby songbird, had flown.

In Martinsville, Mom and Dad prepared funeral arrangements while we stayed at my grandmother's house for the process. During Shelam's illness, my mother had hand-sewn the dress and slip that Shelam would wear to her grave. With great care, she poured her grief into the clothing, stitch by perfect stitch. The mortuary director asked a family member to help prepare Shelam's body, and their work was a testament of love. Shelam's dark hair curled around her unfurrowed brow, while my mother's beautiful garments surrounding her removed the traces of

death. We laid Shelam next to Garnna in Martinsville's South
Park Cemetery.

#

After the funeral, we returned to the Valley. February was bru-
tally cold and gray. Financial and ideological conflicts compounded the grief we suffered. The obligations added to my
father's account from Shelam's care were mountainous. Again,
he implored David for help, but David refused. George continued working a day shift at the sawmill and the machine shop at
night. His disagreement with David festered and spread among
the village, resulting in multiple attempts to frighten or injure
my father.

The lumber industry's growth and the influx of undesir-
able laborers turned the mill areas into a rough-and-tumble
environment that provided an occasion for the first physical
attack against my father. In the logging yard, someone goaded
a simpleton into releasing a semi's load of logs on my father.
Dad escaped the incident by scrambling under the trailer as
thousands of pounds of timber careened into the ditch. These
actions escalated to the use of firearms. The final event involved
a 30 caliber rifle fired from a tree line toward my father as
he drove along the Valley road. The bullet entered the door
frame behind his head, penetrated the vehicle's rear seat, and
exited the back fender. He knew our only option was to leave
Padanaram.

After plowing over seven years and all his finances into the
commune, Dad secured a small home in Bedford and prepared
to flee the village. The fear of hostility and violence was palpable, so we told no one about our plans to escape. A frozen fog
hung in the air the night we left Padanaram. The crunch of the

ice under our feet seemed deafening as the seven of us crept into the car and quietly closed the doors. The mood was tense as the station wagon clambered up the Valley road without the headlights' aid. On reaching State Road 58, Dad stopped to cover the tires with snow chains. As he worked his way around the perimeter, we wiped the condensation from the windows and peered into the forest. Our insides quivered when we noticed a multitude of turkey vultures roosting in the branches of the frost-covered trees encompassing us. Unfazed by the birds' eerie image, Dad returned to the driver's seat, started the engine, and headed into the coming dawn.

CHAPTER 2

Cognizant
1974–1978 (3–7 Years Old)

I DON'T RECALL entering the home on Josephine Street, but I remember waking there. The inception of my memory is that of a lucid dream. A moment of consciousness surrounded by souls I've always known. Faces applied to voices and a sense of belonging. I was safe among sweet people, but there was an underlying current, close to the surface; an engulfing hurt experienced by everyone.

Josephine Street was a frontage road off the well-traveled State Road 39. The businesses erected along its length shielded the homes on the west side of the street from traffic noise, but they also blighted them. The view out of anyone's front door was toward a dumpster, scrap yard, parking lot, or dilapidated structure. Fortunately, everyone's back door opened on hay fields bisected by grassy lanes to disused gravel pits and quarries, and if you walked far enough, you could climb down to the banks of White River.

I slept on a twin bed in a small room that I shared with my sister Carrie. From our berth, we could see a pine-barren spit of damp black ground bordered by a weed-choked fence. Just inside the window, adjacent to my headboard, was a narrow table that supported my sister's record player and provided enough space for me to draw and color pictures. Carrie's bed was a few feet away. The sound of her breathing and the shape of her shoulder in the dim light of the morning were peaceful. Her presence made me feel how a chick must when it's tucked away under a downy wing and sheltered from a chilly rain. Carrie was fifteen, and like most girls of her age, she was in love with love. Her feelings flowed like a fountain; she ambled through each day as if she were the subject of a song played from her well-worn album soundtrack from the movie Sunshine.

#

When Carrie involved herself in my grandmother's Pentecostal religion, she bought me a suit and knee socks and took me with her. I was three years old, and I didn't settle well with the venture for more than a few reasons. The most evident reason was that, beforehand, while waiting on the church bus to pick us up, my brothers climbed into the back of my father's truck to go fishing. It didn't matter where they were going; what mattered was that I wasn't with them.

My grandmother attended Potter's Church; my parents worshipped there before following David. My uncle, Harold Stanger, and his wife Joann, or "Aunt Jobee" as we called her, were also part of the congregation.

Aunt Jobee led the musical portion of the service. She wore horn-rimmed glasses and kept her hair like a coiled beehive atop her head. If not for her hairdo, you wouldn't have noticed her behind the walnut podium. With her eyes closed and one hand raised in worship, she maintained tempo by slapping her hip. She proudly howled at the top of her range as the voices of the congregation joined her. Their sounds were a mixture of natural talent and earnestness that mirrored the sunlight cast through the faux stained-glass windows.

After the song service, I filed out of the sanctuary, among the other children and descended into the church's musty basement; its bowels were rife with the tang of stone, mold, and cut earth. The carpets were usually wet from groundwater, and the teachers warned us of where not to sit or step. Sock-puppet shows were the regular Sunday school fare. Each weekend, a moral battle raged between a plastic head of Jesus - out of scale with his ill-proportioned hands - and a black stocking Devil whose frame was the delicate shape of a woman's hand, faced with a red tongue and jolene eyes. The Devil had flair and character and was always more appealing to watch. He seemed to be the underdog and too smart to lose. Maybe the Devil had plans. Perhaps he was playing a long game and could somehow win. I pined for him to drag Jesus below the blue velvet curtain and return for a solo show. Throughout the entertainment, I could hear shouting and stamping through the tiled ceiling. I could tell old Brother Potter was "under the anointing," as he called the behavior, but it sounded more like a rolling fistfight that my brothers often waged.

Eventually, Brother Potter's row subsided like the end of a spring thunderstorm, and the battered Hammond organ respired. The notes sounded low, like an old man groaning to himself over tragic memories. These undertones were the signal for my release from the Lazarus tomb that was the chapel's subterranean hold. I took the red-carpeted stairs - two at a time - and sprang to the center church aisle with the other kids. The

Sunday morning light, beaming through the stained windows, was in full glory. The sun filled the space in a dazzling display.

The congregation stood, clapping and crooning along with the Hammond - its tune now shed of age and grief. Brother Potter strutted in time upon the pulpit with his punchy face covered in sweat and his unbuttoned suit coat flailing behind him. I imagined that they were singing for me as if I had emerged from a cold crypt, released from death, healed and born again.

A rapturous feeling overtook me as I rounded the corner of the family pew and saw the smiling faces of my grandmother, Carrie, and my Uncle Harold. The reunion washed away the loss I'd felt for them over the previous hour. The congregation rendered a few more songs as the ushers passed the brass offering plates.

Uncle Harold owned an aviator's watch that girded his muscled arm. The timepiece - masterfully crafted in stainless steel with jeweled movements - drove multiple sweeping hands that marked the church service's final minutes and seconds. He must have noticed how I poured over the silver gauntlet; he pulled a pen from his pocket and created - on my wrist - a matching ticker with similar features. For good measure, he added a few hairs and tattoos to my forearms. I couldn't wait to show everyone at home.

Harold "Unck" Stanger

Uncle Harold, or Unck, as I called him, was forty-nine when he pulled me from under my sister's wing and put me on his shoulder. He was rounding the age when a man typically imparts his soul to a grandchild for safekeeping. Unck was also under the misguided assumption that his heritage would end but, fortunately, I was there to remedy the situation.

Unck regularly attended Potter's Church. I believe he tended a spiritual grain, but not wholeheartedly on Sunday mornings, at least not when I was with him.

Unck worked diligently while he was young. By the time we met, he was enjoying the fruits of his labor; he had a quiet home, rental properties, a profitable business, and two pensions. He was fond of expensive toys and shared the best ones with me.

His primary coach was a 1971 Cadillac Coupe de Ville, finished in an elegant burgundy. My first excursion in the Cadillac was on a rainy Sunday morning when he christened me with the title of Copilot and the time-honored distinction of Second in Command. He sat me on his lap to help steer the red ship into any puddle we thought might sink us. We howled with laughter as the muddy spray crashed across the windshield. Aunt Jobee, sitting in the passenger seat, appeared uncomfortable as I exhibited my driving prowess. In fear, she covered her face with both hands, but I swear I could hear her laughing.

Unck's secondary but most prized form of conveyance was the winged type, a red-and-white Piper Cherokee that sported torpedo-shaped "wheel pants." On Sundays, when the sky was bright and Aunt Jobee had to be at church early, Unck, alone, picked Carrie and me up for Sunday school. We delivered Carrie to the chapel entrance and then, with a wink and a nod between us, drove past the parking lot, across Martinsville, and out to the grass airstrip that bordered the old gravel pit. As soon as we pulled off the state road, I scanned the row of exposed wooden hangars, right down to the end, searching for the sleek red nose of the craft. That Cherokee looked like it was moving while sitting. The dart-shaped fuselage and swept-back wings gave it the appearance of an angry wasp, hovering above the ground.

Unck was a veteran pilot and was very thorough in his pre-flight checks. First, we observed the windsock.

Unck asked, "Which way is she pointing?"

"Down!" I exclaimed.

We ran our hands along the craft's body, feeling the skin for damage and the flaps for movement. We recorded the fuel level and inspected the wheels. On completing the exterior audit, we pulled the shining bullet out of the hangar and positioned it toward the grass strip. The examination continued after seating ourselves in the cockpit. We fitted our headsets, checked our microphones, and then signaled the nearest tower with the flight plan.

After recording data and synchronizing the clock with his watch, Unck called out, "Pilot to Copilot. Master switch," and waited for my reply.

I flipped over the red cover of the master switch and turned the toggle to the ON position and responded, "Copilot to Pilot. Master switch ON."

Unck called out again, "Pilot to Copilot. Ignition." I reached up, shaking with excitement, and held down the ignition switch. The knifelike propeller, with its polished nose cap, started its violent rotation. With a few chugs, it disappeared into an animalistic roar that shuddered the aircraft.

I yelled through the headset, giddy with adrenaline, "Contact!"

Taxiing to the top of the grassy runway caused my heart to pound like a bird trapped in hand. Preparing for takeoff, Unck adjusted the flaps and the trim. Slowly, he eased the throttle forward and pulled back on one of the dual controls. Unck released the brakes and let the propeller do its work.

The sun was at our backs. Faster and faster, we rolled with the cornstalks rushing by on each side. The Cherokee felt as if it was being torn apart by the rough ground and the bellowing monster that was the prop. As we bore down toward the face of the gravel pit with the fuselage rattling, the situation seemed terminal. We lifted and shed the cacophony of destruction just short of the gorge as if carried away by angels. With a few sways and a banking climb above the state road, we were in heavenly delight.

After quickly gaining elevation, we leveled off and brought the throttle back. The rising sun to our starboard side cast its presence on the fog that blanketed Martinsville. Here and there, church steeples, grain elevators, and hilltops projected through the mist like watchmen over what lay hidden below.

Unck communicated to the tower and then laughed, looked at me, and said, "Well, we probably shouldn't land until that fog burns off!" He was in his element, soaring, and I enjoyed his happiness. We let the wind carry us eastward to a fly-in diner. The descent to the asphalt landing zone was thrilling. Plummeting from the sky with the treetops rushing by, the sudden rumble of being earthbound again, and the pressure of the harness against our bodies as Unck dropped the flaps felt jeopardous.

After parking the Cherokee, we walked across the tarmac and into the hangar-side diner and ordered an enormous stack of pancakes and a pile of bacon. After filling our bellies, Unck slipped me a five-dollar bill under the table, nodding for me to pay the waitress. My wealth and piloting ability impressed her; she couldn't resist kissing the top of my head.

With a hop, skip, and jump, we repeated the flight procedures and returned to Martinsville. The bright morning light dazzled my eyes. I focused on the fog—stricken by the sun—retreating westward out of the town.

After filling the Cherokee with fuel and tucking it into the hangar, we roared across town in the Cadillac toward Potter's Church. We eased the coupe into the parking lot and listened to the radio while we recounted the previous few hours. Once the churchgoers vacated the building, we pulled around to the front steps and waited for Aunt Jobee and Carrie to exit. Carrie wandered off to ride with a friend while Aunt Jobee headed our way. After closing the door of the De Ville, she looked over her glasses at Unck and pursed her lips.

Turning to look out the window, she questioned his absence, "I noticed you weren't in the pews?"

Unck responded, "There was so much fog; we couldn't land until it burnt off."

Aunt Jobee looked at Unck with a scowl and then down at me with a smile.

#

Whenever we were in his brothers' company, Unck always questioned me, "Who's the best uncle in the whole wide world?"

Missing the joke, I looked into their eyes while doing a buffalo shuffle and responded, "Well, all of you are!" Their laughter released me from my fear of making a social faux pas. They knew I loved Unck. He was more than my mother's brother; he was and continued to be a boy's best friend.

#

Unck eventually received his grandchild. His daughter, Penny, suffered a divorce over accusations of being barren. Shortly after her second marriage, Penny found she was pregnant. The years seem to peel off Unck when he held his granddaughter. Watching him with my new cousin made me aware that he wouldn't need me much anymore. I figured he'd teach her how to copilot and handle the preflight checks. As sad as it made me, I was happy to witness Unck be more pleased than I'd ever seen him.

Sounding

The seven remaining members of our band felt cramped in our modest home; if the weather wasn't certifiably inclement, we spent our time outside. My explorations were nearby, and the most interesting haunt was Mr. and Mrs. Cooper's homestead. Luther and Lola Cooper lived next to us in a house made of limestone. Their large brindle mastiff, Brinson, guarded the property. Geodes, wind chimes, foundry glass scrap, and empty ham cans garnished their windows and sidewalks. A werewolf, featured in a glow-in-the-dark poster harvested from a cereal box, hung above a freezer in their galley kitchen. A painting of dogs playing poker, mounted in a frame above their fireplace, kept them company. They assembled their place of living traditionally (without a bathroom or running water) because Luther believed that "only an animal shits in its own den!" Each dawn, they followed one another outside to a small bathhouse for their morning duties and washing.

The Coopers were a weathered old couple but behaved as if they were untouched by time. Brinson, waning with age, bore numerous scars like badges of honor. It was impossible to look at his copper-and-black striped coat without vividly imagining his adventures. Stories of his escapades were plainly written on his swollen joints and scarred muzzle, but the more painful events seemed hidden behind his tired, chestnut-colored eyes. Those eyes held me with a glow when we met face to face each day in his yard. He let me hang my arm over his withers as we inspected the perimeter of the property.

Mr. Cooper's appearance was strikingly similar to the tall stacks of cinder blocks that surrounded the estate, the primary exception being his bib overalls, white t-shirts, and worn work boots. He kept a silver flattop haircut and a few teeth. His lips, always full of tobacco, seldom parted save for mumbling instructions, spitting, or roaring "bear's ass" to bracket his opinions concerning most of the day's topics. Mr. Cooper shared this signature phrase with the public on a stone plaque mortared into the top of his chimney.

He formed concrete to put food on the table; his hallmarks were blocks, benches, birdbaths, and the occasional grave marker. Mountains of busted block and stone rubble covered the fringe of the construction yard. Despite perpetually cautioning me to avoid the heaps, Mr. Cooper regularly untrapped my feet from the shifting fragments. He readily answered my requests for help by roaring "Augh, bear's ass!" as his callused mitts pulled away brick and hoisted me up by my shoulders.

Mr. Cooper read the sky like the face of a clock. Any sign of rain, too few or too many clouds, or the sun's position in any relation to the horizon, allowed him to peer into the distance, spit, and say, "Better'd head to the porch." This ability often saved him from unnecessary sweating or strenuous exertion.

When Luther ceased laboring, we sat on metal chairs in the shade of the front porch. He drank his beer, lost in thought, while I stared at him, wondering how another human being could appear so like a pillar of limestone. Near the screen door, stacked in wood crates, Mr. Cooper kept little brown bottles of Pabst next to yet another ham can of water for Brinson. I wasn't personally familiar with beer but understood that it was something that adults drank. At least Luther seemed fond of drinking it after a day of dust and sand.

During one of our respites, I asked, "Mr. Cooper, what are you drinking?"

With his voice more gravelly than usual, he replied, "Beer! You want some?"

I accepted his offer, took a sip of the bitter brew, and grimaced.

He rumbled and asked what I thought of its taste by stating, "That's purty good, ain't it?"

I returned my opinion, "Mr. Cooper, that tastes awful!"

Full of pride from the lesson he taught me, he bellowed and laughed, "Augh, bear's ass!"

I, having sampled an adult beverage, felt privileged and ushered into manhood. My first taste of alcohol turned into a fair bit of comedy between us. Every afternoon, I asked, "Mr. Cooper, what are you drinking?"

His response was consistently the same, "Beer! You want some?"

He then slapped his dusty, denim-covered leg, laughed, and roared, "Augh, bear's ass!," as I laughed and bellowed along with him.

Luther used doublespeak like submarines use sonar; he never really said what he meant, hoping to sound another intelligent person who could respond similarly, providing comment or comedy on the situation. Understanding this time-honored second language of men was a challenge, but I reveled in its application, feeling like his peer after grasping its nuances.

#

Mrs. Cooper—short, stout, and spunky—attired herself in polyester slacks, sleeveless plaid shirts, unkempt hair, and horn-rimmed glasses. Although her clothes fit perfectly, the spectacles were never in their correct place on the bridge of her tiny nose. Mrs. Cooper's hands, covered in a lacework of scars and calluses, felt warm and soft on the back of my neck or on my hands when she held them. She spoke with a high-pitched nasal voice, often interrupted by a henlike chuckle. When she communicated with people, she canted her head, placed the top of her wrists on her hips, and stood in apparent wonder as she listened to them speak.

She tended their property and kept many flowers along the roadside masonry fence. Every year, Mrs. Cooper raised an extensive garden adjacent to Waltz's liquor store across Josephine Street. Much to her consternation, drunks frequenting the liquor store crossed the alley to micturate on the vegetables almost every night. She regularly chastised them while shining a flashlight on their rude activity.

The errant urination issues ended one summer night with a loud blast and terrible screaming; Lola loaded a shotgun with rock salt and discharged the contents into some inebriated soul's backside. An uninvolved neighbor called the Sheriff's Department, which dispatched an officer.

On viewing the scene and holding a short discourse with the parties involved, the deputy told Lola, "You can't go around shootin' people, Mrs. Cooper."

The humbled and perforated urinator staggered away, and the lawman returned to his patrol—wearied by trying to dissuade Lola from holding her ground. Instances of people relieving themselves in the alley came to an abrupt halt.

#

Mr. and Mrs. Cooper were the first friends I encountered outside of my family. They were a fixture on the street and were always there when we needed shepherding while our parents had to be away. I never witnessed a cross exchange between them and anyone else, other than someone who could have brought harm to our enclave. Over the few years we lived in Martinsville, our families shared grief, joy, labor, and rest. From whiling away my days with the Coopers, I learned how adults should behave toward a weaker mind who finds themselves out of place or in an unfamiliar environment. They made me aware of how to hold an opinion—and property—and that long patience can end abruptly, possibly in violence.

Want and Acceptance

Day by day, my brothers and I were thick as thieves or thin as specters.

Lamech couldn't get far enough away from me unless we were alone or surrounded by darkness, which was often the case on Saturday nights. Although he jealously guarded all his possessions, he failed to stop me from obsessing over every shining example of his pride, from football trophies to his ruby metal-flake motorcycle helmet.

Joe was my mother's helper; Danny and Lamech teased him incessantly as they figured he was queer for gravitating toward characteristically female activities. If we were hunting or fishing, he was at the edge of the field, making dolls from flowers or corn husks. His only friends were the old ladies at Potter's Church. To us, his most notable activity was that of keeping a clean house. Joe's typical response to the harassment was a warning of sharing his plight with "Mother." If pressed further, he resorted to violence by rocketing one of his stout-heeled shoes at our heads. Joe was tenacious, and I believe the fountain of torment we served him, produced the grit he exhibited in life.

My oldest brother, Danny, was the epitome of a brother; he was fifteen, aloof, and irritable but always in the shadows, ready to provide protection. He did what all boys do; he turned counter to Dad's authority. Figuratively, Dad gave him a lengthy line to run, but Danny—by criminal mischief or ignorant misuse of property—hung himself on it. Danny's adventures entertained us but infuriated Dad.

Carrie was finishing high school and spent a lot of time with her friends from Potter's Church. She was also dating, and we thought it a great comedy to spy on her—through the curtains—as various boys dropped her off at home.

I was too small to keep my brothers' pace and they usually left me behind to sort time by myself. Boredom dictated my schedule. Josephine Street was void of children my age except for two boys, one a few years older and one a few years younger. Mom warned me to stay away from both as the more senior was fond of running me down with his bike, and the other had split my brow with a pipe. The incident with the pipe led to stitches above my eye to seal the wound. My brothers assuaged this pain with a small kaleidoscope. I repeatedly winced in pain while pressing it to either eye, as they howled in laughter at my miserable spectacle. We found great comedy in each other's misfortunes and often tangled ourselves in simple abuses and twisted fights.

If I wasn't at the Coopers', I climbed into dumpsters, crawled through ditches, and explored every old footpath, tree line, gravel pit, and vacant building. There was a lot to study; dead snakes, mulberry trees, frogs, and naval guns on display at the Legion were all vexing. Waltz's liquor store was a major source of entertainment. It was a watering point between Bloomington and Indianapolis, and like a shrinking pool in an arid savanna, its clientele was diverse and entertaining. I encountered local celebrities and individuals creating their infamy. A Coca-Cola vending machine commanded the corner of the building like a glimmering god, filled with sweet nectar. It taunted me. I shoved the few pennies I had into its mouth, but it spit them out; it rejected all my offerings. I wove my small arm through its nether regions, hoping to extract its prize, but failed. At night, its light burned my eyes. I hated it but wanted its love.

Danny piloted his model plane—a Cox-powered P-51 Mustang—from Waltz's parking lot. I lusted over the aircraft, but Danny barred me from touching it. I developed a fascination with Cox engine fuel; it offered heaven in more ways than one. I held the can of gas to my nose, high on the odor and the aerial display, while Danny entertained himself with the flight. I tried to match his aeronautical prowess with my rubber-band-powered balsa airplanes from the IGA, but failed.

#

I loved my brothers, and I longed to be with them, but Mom's enrollment in school made this difficult.

Mom and Dad fought over her desire to do anything but stay at home. He steadfastly believed her paramount responsibility was to maintain the household. She countered his ideology with assertions; she needed to finish high school and wanted to work as a nurse. The nightly arguments subsided once she shot a hearty "Fuck You!" across his bow. My parents never used foul language, and this well-placed munition settled the matter. Mom earned a GED and enrolled at Indiana University to pursue a degree in nursing.

#

Everyone seemed to cope with the loss of Shelam except for Mom; she was often frighteningly distant. With vacant eyes and her face void of character, it appeared as if an invisible hand moved her like a puppet through the day. She suffered from a deep depression, but there wasn't time, resources, or even personal tools to release its pressures. She needed to get away. Maybe improving her education and distancing herself from home might help. As Mom separated herself from the facets of our daily life, I overheard snippets of conversation about sending me to Mamaw's until Mom finished school; due to my age, she wanted to place me under the charge of extended family members.

#

On a gloomy morning in September, Mom pulled me from my bed and coaxed me into the car. With sleep in my eyes, I could still recognize points along the road that revealed we were traveling to my Grandma Stanger's house. When we arrived, Mom shuffled me to the living room, laid me down on the davenport, and covered me with a quilt made from the less worn remnants of old calico dresses. The regulator clock on the wall knocked away in its wood and glass case. Its sound, reminiscent of in utero vibrations, soothed me back to slumber.

I awoke before sunrise to Unck's callused hand on my forehead as he asked, "Do you want some breakfast?"

"Yes!" I replied and followed him through the unlit rooms.

The odor of fried bacon infused the house. In the distance, light—like a beacon of hope—filled the doorway of the kitchen.

Mamaw stood at the stove, wiping her hands and smiling at me, as she affirmed, "You'll want cocoa!"

I happily agreed as I took a seat on a stool between Unck and Uncle Adrian. They regularly joined my grandmother for breakfast, and on this morning, they explained I would join them as long as Mom was going to school. This piece of

information warmed my soul as Mamaw placed a cup and saucer in front of me and filled them both with hot chocolate.
She divvied out plates of fried eggs, bacon, and layers of brown
toast wet with butter. She took her customary position at the
table's side and showed me how to cool and drink the cocoa by
tipping it from the cup and sipping it from the saucer.

#

Mamaw's house was considerably larger than my home on
Josephine Street, and like a mouse in a maze, I explored. To
regulate temperature, plastic sealed two of the unused bedrooms and they were hot or cold, depending on the season.
One chamber acted as a shrine, packed with artifacts from her
sons who served in the Second World War. Silk souvenir pillows
from various military garrisons dressed the chenille-covered
bed. Photographs, faded newspaper clippings, and pale ribbons
adorned the cracked plaster walls. I poured over the coins and
trinkets that littered the top of the mirrored dresser and tried
to wrap my mind around their origin.

Sheet-covered furniture, antique toys, and boxes from the
previous decades filled the second room to its ceiling. A door
in the corner opened to the attic. When I opened it, the odor
of mothballs rolled out into the space. Peeling wallpaper, old
calendars, tin signs, tools, yardsticks, fruit-crate lids, and crum-
bling sheets of newspapers clothed the stairwell. A single tattered cotton string led up the wall and disappeared into the
darkened floor above. I surmised that the string was anchored
to a light somewhere in the shadows. If the mummified line
failed in its purpose, I wouldn't be able to explore the loft as I
was fearful of the dark. The prospect of what could be in that
unknown territory was thrilling, and the possibility of never
discovering what lay there was frustrating.

I pulled on the cord and it gave in my hand. In the upper distance, a ringing click ushered light from a single bright bulb. The swinging illuminated fixture seemed to capture the last vestiges of phantoms leaving the loft. The dusty stairs plaintively sounded under my feet as I elevated my position. The view from the top step revealed more boxes from past ages and a litter of mothballs on the floor.

I tried to search the room, but the dancing shadows and ancestral portraits on the wall piled unease on my shoulders. With terror creeping behind my eyes, I made my way to the darkest far corner, but just short of realizing what lay hidden there, I heard Mamaw calling for me. I was thankful that she'd relieved me from the embarrassment of submitting to my fear. Like an outnumbered gunfighter, I backed slowly from the corner and down the stairs. On reaching the bottom, I pulled the lifeline to the light and returned the attic to darkness. I knew I would return.

#

Like most structures people live in, Mamaw's home was the embodiment of her soul. The struggles and joys that came with raising an extensive family during troublesome times marked the house. The remains of carpeting that once allowed the wealthy to pad through a local sanitarium hid worn wood floors. Before the Depression forced their oldest sons away, they covered the living room walls with a floral print.

Decades previously, when his employer went under due to shrinking finances, Papaw didn't have funds to buy coal for the furnace. Along with other locals, he scavenged lumps of fuel from the rail yard until the night a railroad bulldog shot him. Papaw survived, but the furnace didn't. He replaced it with a secondhand gas burner that still whispered by the front door.

Now, Mamaw's dwelling seemed like a sanctuary, but it was more likely a place of loneliness. The only palpable pulse of the residence was the knock of the wall clock and the creaking of her rocking chair. Nightly, she washed with Dove soap from a porcelain basin, combed her long white hair, dressed for sleep, walked past her children's vacant bedrooms, and knelt beside her bed to pray. My Grandfather's empty berth, smooth and cold, lay adjacent to hers.

#

Mamaw showered me with accolades and honored me with the knightly duty of her rescue. Initially, I questioned her enthusiasm over my qualities, but those frequenting her house agreed with her opinion of me. I remained mildly suspicious until we labored together. That's when I realized I really could shine for her.

During the summer, my prime responsibility was as a sentinel over her garden; according to Mamaw, starlings, grackles, and rabbits plagued it. We observed the crops from the promontory position of her back-porch swing. Usually, we prepared fruit or vegetables while verbally noting the sun's passage across the lawn. Also, we visually scoured the foliage for enemies of the harvest. She had a sharper eye than mine and often noticed the interlopers before the assault. Whenever she cried, "There's a bird in the garden!," I'd immediately drop my colander and advance toward the patch, viscerally shouting and waving my arms to scatter the invaders. I felt a little taller as I trekked back to the portico, but the excitement seemed too strenuous for Mamaw. With both hands, she covered the tears in her eyes and shook uncontrollably.

In the autumn, I carried canning jars from the cellar to the kitchen, where we processed apple butter, beans, and fruit for the coming cold. She told me she needed help and claimed she couldn't see the bubbles from the boil. I stood on a stool for what seemed like hours, staring into the steaming pots and spying for evidence of purification.

Winter passed slowly and comfortably. Mamaw sat in her rocking chair next to the radiant gas stove and rocked me on her short lap. She sleepily rubbed my back with her work-worn hands while we watched her parakeet preen its green feathers. On the list of pleasures a human can record, these moments are written in permanent ink.

#

She had a few friends that visited her. I knew of their expected arrival when Mamaw employed me to set up chairs and a few sawhorses in her bedroom. I don't remember the names or the ladies' faces that called on Mamaw, but I could now recognize them by their stocking-clad legs and leather shoes. The setting was for quilting, and I lay between the structure under the ever-growing cover above me. I watched their hands working needles and thread through cut fabric, lulled by the changing colors and their clucking murmurs.

#

Spring brought hope with the soapy odor of lilacs blowing through the sheer curtains billowing over recently opened windows. After being cooped up over the previous months, we ventured uptown to Kivett's, the local five-and-dime store. Mamaw perused the flat box-bins that stood on wooden floors.

I lingered near the candy counter's glass front, hoping she might notice my yearning for sour cherries and cinnamon balls.

On our return route, we meandered beside the veterans' home. It was a Victorian structure with a detailed porch that wrapped around its extremities. The carnage and refuse of four wars sat in the shade along the perimeter. Old and young men, some missing limbs and others wearing mangled faces, gazed out from the shelter while smoking various tobacco products. I met their eyes, and I couldn't look away.

I wondered if they were friendly like Unck's friends, Jess and Earl, who served together in the Great War. Jess and Earl lived in a tiny shack. It was their residence ever since they returned from France. They never had wives but had black and tan pictures of naked women they must have known. They didn't say much when we visited, but they mumbled a lot. Unck said the war took their hearing. He bought and delivered a paper sack of food to them every Sunday and helped them straighten up the house. I tried to talk with Jess, but he repeatedly shook his head and squinted at me. He kept his mouth closed when he smiled because he had no teeth, and it stretched from ear to ear but looked more like a frown. Both were so thin you could almost see through them. They were small and seemed young, like boys, but their eyes said otherwise.

When the warming days passed into evening, Mamaw and I sat in red metal rocking chairs on the front porch. We monitored the passing traffic and expected my mother's car to be among the procession. The prospect of returning to Josephine Street excited me, and I intently expressed what I wanted to do when I arrived home. Mamaw seemed more interested in the sound of the mourning doves in the area than in my detailed list of activities awaiting me. She kept changing the subject by asking me to listen to them and surmise how many were aloft. She was so enamored of them that she urged me to call them to the yard by directing me to stand next to the rose of Sharon (*Hibiscus syriacus*) and mimic their mournful song. I may have become too chatty in my excitement over my family reunion.

My brothers didn't share my desire to be reunited. Each evening, it seemed as if I was falling further behind them. I had an increasingly smaller stake in decision making. There was no way I could meet them midflight, and I felt like an outsider.

#

Our home was in a sad state when we moved to Martinsville. The roof leaked, and the property needed a new well and septic system. There was a garage, but it was falling in on itself; the first work we tackled was pulling it down. As a four-year-old, I was finally able to help out, so I moved bricks and loaded boards on the fire. We burned the remains of the garage for weeks, and its cracked concrete footing became our outdoor cooking site. A gnarled silver maple tree stood at its western end, and it wasn't uncommon to see a deer carcass or stringers of fish hanging from its boughs. Living under those branches of an evening or weekend afternoon was a way to maintain what we loved about the Valley, and it caressed my earliest memories of wood smoke and dying embers mirrored in the night sky.

We spoke of our time in Padanaram as if it were a badge of honor. Now, the way we were living didn't offer the challenges or rewards from surviving in a wilderness. Dad's few friends from the commune occasionally drifted to our house, having hitched rides from Bedford. They sat under the light of a single bulb in the kitchen, smoking cigarettes and talking of business, societal injuries, and spiritual things. They carried their conversation deep into the night as I fell asleep on my father's lap, and their words found purchase in my subconscious.

#

Like all fathers on Josephine Street, ours returned each evening around 6:30. Hourly schedules were an unwelcome change from our culture in Padanaram. In the commune, everyone was near, and no one had to leave. We were with our family at each meal, and we could watch or even help our parents work. Now we were in increasingly divided subcultures.

Dad was the gravitational center of our universe. Though scattered throughout the day, we drifted to alignment when he was present. We revered Saturday evenings and Sunday mornings; they provided the hours when Dad was available. We loved being with him, and all pined for his recognition, but there wasn't enough time to accommodate everyone's interests. Fortunately, his noise before dawn woke me and attuned me to his schedule. I enjoyed having his undivided attention as I sat on his lap in the scant glow of a table lamp. The smoke from his cigarette in the ashtray rose in delicate tendrils toward the light. He drew pictures for me on the back of unopened mail while he sipped from a coffee cup. We talked about things I found in dumpsters, frogs in the old quarry, and flying in Unck's airplane. One morning, I asked him about my name; all the mispronunciations and comedic jabs wearied me. He recounted his dream from before I was born and consoled me with the idea it was essential and given by God.

If Dad didn't have to work on a Saturday, once the sunrise filled the windows, he and I moved to my brothers' room where Dad taunted them to wake by singing "The Battle of Kookamonga." He refused to allow anyone to sleep late as he had a multitude of tasks that needed to follow a schedule.

After a breakfast of oatmeal and scrambled eggs, a boiler-plate special in our household, we raced, tripping and shoving each other for a prime position in the back of Dad's truck. His hauler was a bright point in our life in Martinsville. He purchased it in new condition for a "great deal" from a local dealership. The Ford sat in the lot for over a year because its pea-green finish was unappealing. We loved the rig because it was superior to the car we'd used to flee from Padanaram, and we could all ride in it with no one having to sit on another's lap.

Dad had a prodigious work ethic that made us uncom-fortable; he usually continued his activities past any measure of reason. Even when he claimed to be resting or taking time off, he finagled a final touch on some bit of labor. Dad's list of chores always comprised helping someone, fishing, and forag-ing. Sometimes, all those missions merged at one location, but we rambled across multiple counties more often than not. We repaired earthmoving equipment on the sides of hills, cleaned out sheds for elderly friends, and visited old stewards of my father who could no longer leave their homes.

After completing Dad's duties, we meandered out to Larry Hess's fish hatcheries to squander what remained of the day until climbing back into the truck's bed. We viciously fought over the wheel wells but as usual, the smaller of us sat with our backs to the cab where flecks of windborne sand and grit pecked at our faces. The feeling of defeat was not lasting. When the sun gave way to the moon, and our ears ached from the cold, we all huddled for warmth in the bed's bottom. We each took our turn shuffling to the center of our cluster while the others pro-vided cover. In the truck, exposed to every imaginable element, we watched the changing panorama of southern Indiana. We offered opinions on what we saw and what we were doing. The week's previous separations and anxiety fell away from us like the disappearing road behind the tailgate. Under the uninterrupted sky, we forgave transgressions and restored egos. We felt indomitable while hurtling toward a common destination with a shared burden, and I felt whole, connected, and safe.

CHAPTER 3

Anderson
1979 (8 Years Old)

IN THE SPRING of 1979, Dad received a promotion at Universal Tool and Engineering in Indianapolis. To be closer to his employer, he bought a ranch house in one of many 1960s subdivisions bordering substantial farmlands in west Anderson, Indiana. In June, when Mom graduated from nursing school and found a job as a licensed practical nurse in Noblesville, Dad sold our home on Josephine Street, and we moved north.

Moving away from Martinsville troubled me. Several hurtful changes had me figuring more were on the way. We left behind the most influential people in my life. Carrie stayed in Martinsville and lived with Mamaw, and Unck—along with the Coopers—was more than an hour's drive from us. I was eight years old and could look after myself, but it stung not to enjoy their presence.

Beyond the geographic separations and uprooting of foundational connections, minuscule facets of life slipped out of position. They made life feel washed and civilized, unlike the marrow-filled substance of my previous eight years. While Danny and Joe transported furniture to our new quarters, a car blindsided them and destroyed our green truck. To replace the vehicle, Dad purchased an Oldsmobile sedan and didn't permit us to wear our field clothes in it unless towels covered the seats. Our foraging and fishing expeditions all but ceased.

Dad labored at Universal Tool from Monday through Saturday, and Mom worked third shift so she slept at odd hours throughout the day. Sunday mornings became bizarrely different. We used to deliver papers with Danny and Joe or visit family and friends; now, Mom and Dad started going to church. Shortly before moving to Anderson, I heard my parents discussing Mamaw's trepidation about us leaving Martinsville. To end our tenure there on a pleasant note and console Mamaw, Mom and Dad attended Potter's Church on our final Sabbath in town. During the service, my parents experienced a "movement of the Spirit" and felt the need to devote their lives to God. This spiritual reawakening pulled on them to explore Pentecostal churches in our new hometown. While they sampled Anderson's religious opportunities, we boys stayed home and occupied ourselves with a fresh color TV.

#

My brothers and I didn't particularly appreciate changing schools or losing friends. Being outsiders in a new community came with the expected amount of fear. Fortunately, summer was in full swing, and returning to school was only a distant threat.

There was a magnificent opportunity for me. The neighborhoods surrounding our home were like large nurseries that housed masses of potential companions, and the endless natural landscape that hemmed the western horizon was ripe for exploration. From the front yard, I observed packs of kids roaming the fields and traversing the wooded distance. My challenge was assimilating into the established clans. My struggle didn't last long. One afternoon, while unpacking boxes in the garage, Dad nudged me in the arm and nodded toward a ruddy kid in a blue windbreaker standing at the driveway's edge. The boy watched me, awkwardly shifting his weight from one foot to the other, waiting to be engaged. It was clear he required an introduction so I walked up to him and introduced myself. He called himself Whitey and asked if I wanted to walk around the neighborhood. We headed North and took a turn into the addition. We acquainted ourselves by pontificating on points of pride and found that we shared more than a few common interests.

"I caught six frogs."

"I'm pretty good at drawing pictures."

"I like Farrah Fawcett."

"My brother's got a motorcycle."

"I've got a GI Joe collection."

"Do you like KISS?"

"Yeah. I stayed awake until two in the morning one time."

Since there was enough substance between us to merit a friendship, we decided to have one. I quickly bonded with Whitey; he was the first peer I'd met who could speak in full sentences, didn't breathe through his mouth, and wasn't interested in swinging sticks at my head or running me down with a bike.

His family, recently moved from Illinois, settled in a two-story house on the addition's backside. There wasn't much difference between my home and Whitey's, but the vibe was distinct. The way his parents took time to be together, focusing on having fun rather than doing labor, was foreign. Other than making the occasional joke when he got home from work, my dad was all business, whereas Whitey's dad was comedic and sang folk songs. My friend and I watched as his dad set up an in-home studio where he'd play around, reliving memories made while laying tracks with his friends from college. Whitey's family seemed like a Vaudeville troop, into music and artistic culture. For Friday night entertainment, they acted as the audience for activities such as elaborately memorized skits Whitey and I studiously developed. Joan, Whitey's mother, gushed praise and directed our enterprises from a reasonable distance while Whitey's dad, Whitey Sr., backed us with instrumental guitar tunes. Whitey's sister, Rose, was a few years older and made sport of us, but under her proud surface, you could feel that she loved her little brother.

Whitey decorated his room with posters of album covers and Frank Frazetta art. A swanky console stereo with a gold finish commanded attention as it was his most notable possession, outside of his action figure collections. We spent a lot of time on his shag carpet listening to KISS, staging scenes with his Kung Fu Grip G.I. Joes, and tracing *Conan the Barbarian* comics. As the summer progressed toward the autumn semester, we assimilated into a smattering of boys hailing from multiple residences along Lone Oak Road. Still, he and I remained a close team.

#

Our first day at our new school offered me a new promise; Danny, Joe, Lamech, and I would ride the same bus to a single destination. This change was a departure from our diverse schedule in Martinsville with its segregated elementary, junior high, and high school.

The sky was still dark when the bus's flashing stop sign gave notice up the hill. We watched its halting progression toward our driveway. When the squealing brakes eased the yellow whale to a halt in front of us, we tramped up the steps and made our way down the aisle to the few partially occupied bench seats. Like the solitary combative buck behind a herd of lesser deer, Danny slowly followed our file, observing our surroundings, and took the back seat, attempting to ignore an incredibly irritating noise.

The first thing I heard—that anyone heard—on boarding the bus was a sophomore named Kenny Keenhound. He wore an Army surplus field jacket that smelled like an ashtray full of piss, and his acne competed with his unkempt stubble from a low-talent summer haircut. With an unlit cigarette bouncing between his lips, he spewed brazen obscenities at the other passengers and us. When he flipped Lamech's ears and slapped Joe's books out of his arms, I knew what would happen.

From the corner of my eye, I saw Danny rise from his position. I glanced at him and saw that his face was white and his eyes were glassy, almost teary, as was typical when bombarded with a fit of rage. His chin jutted out with the corners of his lips drawn downward with laser-direct hatred. Roiled, he stalked toward Kenny like a panther. I cast my view at Kenny, whose crooked mouth was in such high gear he was clueless about the menace drifting up the aisle, filling the space behind him. Danny swayed to his left, drawing back a rock-shaped fistful of new pencils, and drove a haymaker straight into the side of Keenhound's head. The impact slammed Kenny against the foggy window. Kenny's skull bobbed around on its pivot until he focused on Danny, who was shaking with fury, standing above him.

Danny growled through clenched teeth, "Don't fuck with my brothers!"

Blood flowed from Keenhound's temple; a fractured pencil point held the wound open.

Kenny dabbed his palm against his head, looked at his crimson-covered hand, and cried incredulously, "You stabbed me with a pencil!"

Danny's lips were still pale as he spit, "Don't fuck with my brothers!"

He crept backward and returned to his seat. His eyes locked in position as if burning holes through Keenhound's skewered, scrunched-up face. Kenny looked for support among his cronies but couldn't find it. The kids on the bus remained anxiously quiet.

Patting his bleeding wound, he vocalized his disbelief, "He stabbed me with a pencil?"

Danny's fits of rage chilled me to the bone. He rarely weathered remarks or actions leveled against him. If he took offense, all traces of rational thought escaped him. Whereas an average person's reptilian brainstem offers options for fight or flight, Danny's basal ganglia routed straight to combat and, like a battleship, he turned broadside and fired all the guns at once. I'd experienced his wrath and knew too well to play away from it. Keenhound didn't understand he had insulted Danny by pestering us, so Danny did him the favor of making him painfully aware. From that point forward, Keenhound lowered his eyes and leaned out of the way every time Danny came down the aisle.

#

As a junior that year, Danny joined the Lapel football team and maintained his position despite his frustration with the school's lengthy string of losses. He came from the Martinsville

Artesians, who seldom lost a Friday night fight. It was a thrill to watch him running as an outside linebacker and crashing through the scrimmage line under the field lights on crisp autumn nights.

Joe and Lamech were in the marching band. I was proud to see them having fun with their recent friends in the south end of the aluminum bleachers. I preferred the company of peers and an unobstructed view of the cheerleaders from a vantage point under the stands.

Mom and Dad eventually joined the Band Boosters and Lions Club, and were also Scout troop leaders. They relished participating in civic activities. They set a moral example, and we learned how to dedicate ourselves to success. I enjoyed being together in these institutions, but the quality of our moments felt fragmented compared to our weekends in Martinsville.

#

My parents settled on joining a United Pentecostal parish on the east end of Anderson near Shady Side Park. On a Monday evening, they sat us down to tell us they had found a "home" in that church, and we would accompany them, not just that coming Sunday but to all events in the foreseeable future.

Telling us this, six days ahead of time, made me think they were breaking the news gently and allowing us space to get our affairs in order. Danny talked his way out of going; therefore, the lucky bastard escaped a session of fitting dress clothes and plastic dress shoes at the mall. I bucked at the plan. Since I now had a bunch of friends to run with, the prospect of killing a Sunday with churchy kids in a musty basement was an abominable insult to my childhood nature and a total waste of my day.

Sunday arrived with a feeling of dread. Joe went willingly, but Dad forced Lamech and me into the Oldsmobile's back seat, sweating in our thick polyester church clothes that were as breathable as trash bags. The odd brother out, Joe, loved any excuse to wear his Sunday best.

#

We pulled into the church's gravel parking lot—nowhere near as manicured, orderly, or uniform as the Potter's Church lot. The chapel lacked the symmetry, grace, and respectability one would usually associate with such an edifice. I estimated the flagstone exterior rivaled the crudeness of the tomb Jesus crawled from after being crucified. The mural of Jesus's resurrection above the baptismal tank behind the pulpit was consistent with the shoddily constructed building. The amber windows, like arrowslits on an old castle, grudgingly allowed a scant light that couldn't reach more than a few feet along the blood-colored pews. A cold green glow from fluorescent lamps screwed to the ceiling replaced the missing illumination.

The structure was scary, dark, confining, and stale. Crypts and cemeteries were more elegant. Our new "church home" was a fortress keeping the perceived darkness of the world at bay. The leaders of this sect had a fear that echoed in their building and their teachings alike. They followed the Bible to the letter, and they tailored their culture to match one that was foreign, thousands of years old, and woefully misinterpreted at that.

Once again, they sequestered me in the cellar with a gaggle of kids who genuinely looked like they enjoyed being there. This establishment offered felted cutouts to portray the birth, life, death, and resurrection of Jesus; Potter's Church, at least, used sock puppets. I yearned to sit upstairs next to my parents as the environment below seemed more akin to the series of *Twilight Zone* episodes I warily watched.

I tried communicating my contempt for being confined in the creepy basement with weird kids for dumb activities. After more than a dozen uncomfortable conversations, I think Mom told Dad to relent. Absolved from subterranean instruction, I returned to the surface with my parents and brothers. This moment was one of the first times I felt they recognized and heard me.

#

One Sunday night, as the pastor railed on about the rapture and the tribulations that were coming as God's vengeance, I quietly thumbed through the concordance of Dad's Bible. I found my name on the second page—"Amalek: Warlike; dweller in the vale." I followed the citations throughout the Old Testament. Dread settled over me when I figured out Dad gave me the name of an evil king who God wanted snuffed from existence.

Since the only accepted form of verbal noise during the service was "Amen" or "Praise God," I silently nudged Dad with my elbow and pointed to the definition. I hoped he'd assuage my panic. I don't think he realized the depth of unease running through me when he firmly nodded.

Dad understood everything in the Bible associated with Amalek. He felt he had no choice but to give me the name imposed on him by some mysterious godlike presence from a nightmare years before I was born. Naming me was not his decision, nor was it his option to change it; bothered by it, he tried to hide it by making it my middle name.

I didn't understand. Why was I named after something that God viciously hated? I knew it came from Dad's dream, but why me? Why was I tagged before birth with such a cruel identity?

The tirade the minister spewed created fearful imagery that sank into my fertile mind. I grew concerned about escaping this predicted horror and listened intently for a resolution.

After the organist coerced the first mournful bars from the Hammond, the pastor began his graceful plea to the congregation, "He that believeth the Son hath everlasting life: and he that believeth not the Son shall not see life; but the wrath of God abides on him." He continued:

> Not everyone who says to me "Lord, Lord," will enter the kingdom of heaven, but only he who does the will of my Father who is in heaven. Verily, verily, I say unto thee, except a man be born of water and of the Spirit, he cannot enter the kingdom of God. That which is born of the flesh is flesh; and that which is born of the Spirit is Spirit. For the time has come for judgment to begin at the house of God; and if it begins with us first, what will be the end of those who do not obey the gospel of God?

Then the pastor called everyone to the front to confess sins and pray for the Holy Ghost's transformative powers. Like animals, late for Noah's Ark, some fled the pews for the pulpit and fell on their knees. Their open weeping softened those with more hardened hearts until they filed down the aisle to join the crowd, where they crumpled and moaned.

I looked to the white-haired elders who undoubtedly rested under the shelter of redemption. They lifted their hands, bowed their heads, and spoke in gibberish I couldn't understand.

I couldn't reconcile the pastor's message of grace with what I read just moments before. I wanted to receive deliverance like the mass of humanity at the altar. I needed to feel the assuredness that the pastor and those behind him must be feeling. I craved freedom from inevitable calamity, but how could I attain it? Being marked as evil before birth, surely no number of godly deeds in my life would allow me into the Rapture and avoid enduring the nightmare of punishing circumstances called the Tribulation.

I didn't believe I had what it would take to live as reverently as Mom and Dad, the church leaders, or anyone who lived the way God demanded. I failed to see beyond this fear. The sum of my reasoning was dire. I would have to endure all the horrible events the Bible predicted. I would not be part of my parents' salvation; I would have to fend for myself in the coming apocalypse without God's help.

I wished I hadn't been born.

#

My conflict with the religious supernatural combined with the popular culture that warned of a nuclear holocaust led to a fascination with preparing for the apocalypse. I voraciously read Boy Scout and surplus military manuals. Wherever I went, I noted avenues of escape, hiding places, and potential shelters. I created lists of necessities for multiyear survival and practiced the art of camouflage. I became a proficient, prolific builder of forts and makeshift weapons. I believed God destined me to lead a dangerous existence, so I pondered which of the females in my class would be fit for repopulating the earth. I pictured myself being the male protagonists in the sci-fi movies and television shows I watched—the adventures and epic love stories between two characters with unparalleled prowess and bravery. While I knew the girls I liked didn't like me, I figured that shaping myself into someone with the mental and physical aptitude to withstand a world-ending cataclysm might make me suitable for a pretty girl's love.

#

The church rhetoric was increasingly troubling. They laid out a lengthy list of activities and facets of everyday living unacceptable to Christianity. My recently gained companions and my most enjoyable vices met with disapproval. The elders deemed my collection of thrift store 45s, comic books, and fantasy art posters satanic, and my passion for drawing was under scrutiny. They cast a shadow on most anything that brought pleasure.

Even though I firmly believed I would burn in Hell forever, I worked to stack up positive measures that might allow me to pass into Heaven. Each night, before I drifted off to sleep, I prayed for the security of my family. I pitched my records, art albums, and the sketch pads I purchased with cash from raking leaves and shoveling snow. I tried to avoid my buddies, and I studied the red Bible Carrie bought me when we attended Potter's Church.

My efforts to live a godly lifestyle did little to soothe my fear of eternity. I was progressively empty and lacking any joy. All my friends except Whitey eventually stopped coming to my door. It tortured me when he asked me to clarify why I wasn't doing what I used to do. Before, we'd traded Frazetta publications, comics, and rock 'n' roll 45s, reveling in our extensive collections. I didn't want to explain why I had thrown all my favorite items away; my attempts to defend my actions left him stunned and incredulous, but he remained my friend.

My self-imposed Bible studies were a torment. I critiqued the six pages of pallid pictures of ancient life and wished Frank Frazetta had crafted them. I recognized without a doubt that that era would have been dirty and harsh. The acts and events described in the Bible were graphic and disturbing. In a fit of jealous rage, Cain murdered his brother Abel with nothing but a stone. David, king of the Hebrews, watched his neighbor's wife taking a bath; he lusted after her, impregnated her, and then sent her husband to the front lines of a battle to kill him. Saul, another king of the Hebrews, consorted with a witch to foretell his future. To protect his guests, a Levite threw his daughter out to a mob that ravaged her to death. Then, the father dismembered her body and spread it around the countryside. Rape, murder, jealousy, contests with fire and wild beasts, and the putting out of eyes were common. The publishers sterilized the illustrations into a midcentury hodgepodge, to not irritate the tender sensibilities of easily offended religious people. I knew they whitewashed the images with untruth if not outright deceit. Beyond this, the rest of the pages seemed like a boring genealogy of foreign names. I skipped over the rules and regulations and focused on the exciting portions of inhuman strength, sex, and destruction. I ended my readings in Revelation, hoping to divine my fate.

#

I took to the woods and fields not so much like John the Baptist on his God-given mission to clear the way for Jesus Christ, but like Cain, marked by God and banished from his tribe to wander the world.

I trusted nature. I learned that its lineage reached back before man trampled and despoiled it. Flora and fauna brought no curse, and according to my Bible, it was the last agreeable life that God created. One fruitful day, I retreated from the house across the field to the west. I clambered through the remnants of rusty barbed wire that, ages ago, failed to contain a couple of hundred acres of isolated forest. After pushing through the brambles, incurring numerous cuts and snags, I beheld a towering beech tree. Mayapples, bleeding hearts, and papery amber leaves blanketed its footing. I put my right hand to the gray trunk and, thinking to wrap my arms around it, slid my left hand across its once smooth bark—now marred with more than a century of carved initials—and pressed my ear to its surface. Even if there had been ten of me circling its torso, we wouldn't be able to encompass its dimension. I turned my head to look up to the treetop and saw what looked like a multitude of eyes covering its height and breadth. Its uppermost branches, flecked with quivering golden leaves, waved in the wind.

I realized the breeze that tore at my jacket as I crossed the half mile of corn stubble and clay couldn't penetrate the copse of trees surrounding me. I backed away from the giant, entranced by its physical stature, and tried to imagine its age and all the events its black eyes must have witnessed.

I felt like a fool when I glanced to mark my entry point; I'd crushed a thirty-foot strip of wildflowers, leaving a trail any blind person could follow. Searching for a less destructive approach, I noticed a web of paths, devoid of vegetation. I'd read about natives tracking silently through the woods, and I picked this opportunity to practice my ability at that skill. I crouched low, balancing on the outsides of my feet, and stalked heel-to-toe between the plants and deadfall until I made it to the nearest trace. The path I found was walnut-colored and softened by more deer traffic than anyone could measure. I touched the concavity of the tracks and tried to surmise how long ago their author pressed them. I knew I wasn't alone in the forest and understood that I'd have to be quieter if I wanted to see any of the things that lived here.

I kept the path down a slope toward the heart of the woods where old giants had collapsed. Creeping water rotted their foundation and pooled in the craters evacuated by upturned roots. I continued drifting down the trail where tracks wove through the scattering of moldering trunks and at places crossed them, leaving yellow scars. The traces dissipated, peppering an expanse of mud that surrounded a glacial bog.

I wanted to close on the lagoon without getting stuck. I conducted my way to a fallen timber and crawled along the log to where it sank in the pool. Through my reflection, it amazed me to see fairy shrimp weaving below the surface. I remembered Josephine Street and the dissatisfaction I had when my mail order of sea monkeys (brine shrimp) hatched and appeared nothing like the happy family of aliens pictured in the advertisement. I felt even more duped when I realized I'd wasted money on livestock I could have freely obtained from any woodland pond. I submerged my hand and pulled out a large specimen. It wriggled in the teaspoon of water trapped in the folds of my palm. Feeling I'd just done something hurtful, I quickly returned it to its universe.

I eased back into an adjoining mass of branches. Suspended above the center of the depression, I looked up through the hole in the canopy and watched a skiff of ash-colored clouds rapidly crossing the white sky. I felt like I'd found a special place. I also thought this could make a decent haven for me while God's Horsemen focused on raping and pillaging the other humans damned to hell.

The sky gradually darkened, and wind licked at the water. I made my way back to the deer trail and followed it in a meandering direction toward home. It crossed from the woods to the field where a tree had grown through the barbed-wire fence and snapped the corroded metal. I pressed my feet in the track to not crumple last summer's weeds and stepped out into the gale. I felt the woodlands calling me to return as I looked homeward and spied the first yellow lights illuminated in defiance of the night settling. By the time I entered my driveway, it was dark but not so dark as to hide Carrie's Chevette.

#

I pushed open the front door and saw Carrie standing in the dining room. She was having a fun time slinging sarcasm with Dad and Danny. Lamech and Joe joined in, too. Mom smiled while she busied herself with cooking a skillet full of Salisbury steak. I sidled next to Carrie and wrapped my arms around her hips. Her goose-down vest smelled of perfume, and her feathered amber hair fell around her shoulders.

She said, "Hey, Bubby," and returned the affection. She wasn't staying for a meal; she visited us on her way to another date with Ted. Ted was the brother-in-law of one of my mom's coworkers. He and Carrie were seeing each other almost every weekend and seemed serious about their relationship.

We all were excited to see Carrie. Like Dad, she glued us together, but in a way that caused you to want to cater to each other. Rooms were warmer and brighter when she was in them. Food tasted better. The air was sweeter. Worry rolled away like water on duck feathers, and peacefulness settled in your soul. You could anger her, but it wasn't a fit of fury that forced you to shrink. It was an exhibition that affirmed that she was harmless, and it made you want her and want to be loved by her. When wrought, she'd stand with a defiant posture, flag the room with an extended finger, roll her eyes skyward—not entirely directing her wrath at you—and unleash a diatribe that always began and ended with, "I'm sorry!"

#

A few weeks later, Carrie and Ted announced their engagement; Carrie moved from Martinsville to our home in Anderson to prepare for their wedding the following autumn. Once again, we shared a room, but she didn't sleep there often. Carrie started two jobs in Edgewood, the burg nearest us, where she worked at a hardware store and the locally famous Edge Inn. She spent her weekends with Ted, and I seldom saw her but heard her quiet footfalls in the night as she crept to her bed. In peace, I listened to the familiar sound of her breathing. I turned my thoughts toward Martinsville, where now the Coopers' windows were dark, and Brinson prowled from moon shadow to moon shadow, lifting his head at each pause, monitoring the night air for foreign encroachment. Unck, Aunt Jobee, and Mamaw were surely resting. I imagined a fog creeping from creek branches and forests to the flat parts of town, stealing its way between houses and barns to cover all sleeping things. My eyes followed the mist down State Road 37, between the river and cornfields, until I couldn't see anything but blackness.

#

The Thompson family lived behind us; they were a middle-class household with two boys, Mark and Milton. They had a two-story home with an in-ground pool and owned a Betamax video player. Daily, the boys beat the hell out of each other, frequently fighting over a three-wheel ATV that they abused mercilessly. They were both loud and prone to tantrums, but the younger, Milton, had a rage that unhinged at the drop of a feather, so most kids stayed away from him. I'm not sure how Lamech and I gained their friendship, but we received regular invitations to join them in the pool and watch movies in the evening. Although swimming sounded like a pleasant time, it was more like a morning of drown-proofing with Lamech and Mark estimating how long they could get away with holding Milton and me under the water. It was silent torture; they were quiet with their efforts as Mrs. Thompson, glamorously bronzing her oiled skin in the sun, refused distraction.

Around this stage, a shift occurred between Lamech and me. Admittedly, we had our brotherly brawls, but I felt we covered each other's backs. We built models together, helped each other with chores, and I was his companion when we went into uncharted territory. The tipping point of our fracture took place on the front lawn of the Thompson estate. After watching Sylvester Stallone's victory over Carl Weathers in *Rocky II*, Mark and Lamech fitted Milton and me with boxing gloves to recreate the final scene. After they tied our gloves, I expected Lamech to be my Mickey, but instead of standing behind me, he made his way to Milton's corner of the yard where he and Mark pulled Milton's trigger and spurred him to pummel me into submission. After a few failed bouts, I chewed at my gloves' laces and dropped them at my feet. Feeling betrayed, I walked away. Milton followed me to the street, driving multiple rounds into the back of my head and kidneys. Milton didn't need to knock the wind out of me; Lamech carried it with him to his corner.

After that day, I steered away from Lamech but didn't have to veer far; he released the vestiges of his childhood that had fascinated me and wanted to be alone. He was proceeding into junior high, and by his actions, clarified that there was nothing between us but shared names.

#

There was a freestanding metal cabinet in our garage that I viewed as a shrine; it kept my fathers' and brothers' once prized possessions. The doors rattled when moved on their hinges. The garment bar supported my paternal grandfather's worn Levi's jacket with woven wool liner, its collar and cuffs frayed from a generation of use. Next to the denim coat was the rubber logging slicker Dad wore in the commune when it rained. Above the clothing, on a rack, was Lamech's first motorcycle helmet.

In Martinsville, when Lamech wasn't near, I pilfered the helmet from his bedpost and put it on my head, imagining I appeared akin to Evel Knievel. I practiced with it while stunt riding on Josephine Street until just before Lamech arrived home from school. I always returned the gem to its resting place, hoping he wouldn't notice my sweat on the band. One day, I misjudged his arrival time. The bus rolled alongside me as I rapidly pedaled toward a ramp. From the corner of my eye, I could see the pleasure on the kids' faces; they must have been thrilled by my spectacle. I increased speed, still conscious of my public. They were in rapture now, my jump a mere yard away. I launched into the air—for what seemed like minutes—and came to a side-skidding halt, facing my people, and raised my arms in victory. Panting and proud, I scanned the windows, marveling at my laughing audience, until I noticed a face in one window was not overjoyed. That face belonged to Lamech. He didn't look pleased; he looked angry. He was furious. Fear froze me in place as I watched him tear down the aisle and jettison himself from the door. He charged toward me, and as I recoiled from the coming assault, he wrapped his arms around the helmet to pull it from my skull. He wrenched and pried, growing angrier, failing to realize I'd securely buckled it under my chin. My hands flailed to release the D-rings that now functioned as a garrote. Dragging me through the gravel driveway tired him; he let loose of my helmet-clad cranium and, with a knee, drove his weight into my exposed belly. He panted, roared, and slammed his fists on my sternum until I released the buckle. Growling, he ripped his crown from my head and stormed into the house.

I still viewed the helmet with lust. Its glitter-flake base flashed through the thick ruby topcoat. Three remaining snaps held the smoked bubble-face shield in position. Its silky nylon strap, with its two D-rings, draped over the shelf's edge and seemed to call me. Still feeling a twinge of fear, I drew it from its lair and squeezed it over my ears. I rolled my head around to feel its weight again. I pulled it off and thumbed my nail at the multitude of scratches in the gel coat and wished I needed it.

Behind the jackets, leaning against the back, was Lamech's air rifle! He must have recently cleared out his room. If it was in the locker, it was fair game for anyone, so I grasped the cold steel barrel and lifted it from the shadows. It was a bolt-action pump, Crossman 760. It chambered BBs and shaped lead pellets. It was a modern extravagance compared to the decades-old Daisy BB gun I inherited when Lamech received the Crossman in Martinsville. The Daisy couldn't knock over a pop can from ten feet, but the Crossman readily punched through them. I marveled at its purposeful lines and racked the bolt to the rear, inspecting the chamber's function. I grasped the plastic fore-grip and actuated it to fill the reservoir. I pulled the trigger and released the charge; its familiar sound triggered memories of target practice with Lamech. I shouldered it to check its sights. The 760 would make an excellent addition to my survival stash of surplus Army pouches, tools, and sundries.

#

Carrie and I shared a birth month. She always made it a point to make sure we enjoyed ourselves, and this July was no different. She gifted clothes, but I wasn't interested in western shirts; I just wanted her attention. Knowing this, she assured me we would go to a movie for our birthday. I was excited until she came home with her friends from Martinsville and announced that we would see *Urban Cowboy*. By this summer, her love for John Denver had set like the sun, and the new star of her orbit—besides Ted—was John Travolta. We packed into her two-door Chevette and headed east into Edgewood and further into Anderson. We attended the latest showing, and I slept through most of it. Carrie roused me at the end, and we made our way back to her car. She let me sit in the passenger seat next to her. The breath of night air through the windows, as much as the hour, subdued the previous atmosphere. My head bobbed, weighted by sleep.

When we stopped for the traffic light in Edgewood, Carrie rubbed my chest to wake me. "It's midnight." she said, "Happy Birthday, Bubby."

I looked at the clock and at her eyes; she was radiant when she smiled. It was midnight; I realized it was my birthday. Images of the cherry cake Mom would bake for me flashed through my mind, and the prospect of my birthday falling on a Saturday hailed good fortune.

I quickly came to myself under her gaze and said, "Thanks!" Although it was cool in the car, I was warm. She had a way of making me feel that way.

#

Carrie and Ted married in November. They purchased a farm west of us, in Bakers Corner, and it became a resort for our family. The easiest path to them was over Strawtown Road, and it was a pleasure to observe the undulating expanse of agriculture and hamlets along the way. Our weekly visits opened avenues into activities that had gone fallow since leaving Martinsville. We walked the fields adjacent to the homestead to pull weeds, remove rocks, and scour for arrowheads. We cleaned out the barn loft for storing straw, tore down old grain sheds, and mowed the lanes that crisscrossed the property. Ted built a farrowing house and transplanted a few sows and a boar from his parents' stock. By the following spring, we were notching piglet ears and cutting their teeth and testicles. Cleaning pens was as expected but watching a herd of miniature pink oinkers running hot laps around the shed made it worthwhile. Observing the wheat harvest from the combine's cab was cathartic, and playing in the mounds of uniform grains, destined for the elevator, felt rewarding. The golden hue of the seeds churned genetic memories of wealth and security.

After a few months of marriage, Carrie was swelling and walking with a maternal glow that caused my parents to radiate. The expectant addition to our family brought out qualities in Mom and Dad I'd rarely witnessed. They were joyful. Dad worked fewer hours and dusted off old friendships. He bought new cane poles for all of us, and we fished, coming or going, on Morse Reservoir's banks. He made things out of wood and showed me crafts he'd learned as a boy and while living in Padanaram. We assembled a fish trap to sink in the meadow creek, and soon I was catching more wrigglers than anyone, a cherished mantle to wear. Before the wedding, Mom recovered her sewing machine from Mamaw's and artfully crafted Carrie's bridal gown. Now, she ran fabric at a withering pace, turning out clothes for baby boys and girls to cover either outcome. Mom and Dad were nesting, along with Carrie, and it was a beautiful spectacle.

#

Danny graduated that spring, and under Dad's tutelage, was apprenticing as a machinist. He wasn't home much, but he'd always been a rover. Danny owned a purple Nova coupe with a white fabric top and mag wheels. When he rolled into the driveway, it was like a knight returning from a crusade. In reality, he was usually with his high school love, Laura, who he planned to marry in the coming autumn.

Danny was kind to me. I was always excited to see him and showed my affection by trying to land solid punches on his arms and gut. Feigning a serious sparring match, he took a combative posture and swung wide reaches to slap my temples. Our games ended with him gaining a better position to wrap his palm around my forehead and clamp my head under his arm. For reasons unknown, he invariably sealed his victory with a well-timed fart.

He and Dad still sparred, and it wasn't always a friendly competition. Dad didn't cater to Danny's temper, and Danny never backed down. I witnessed their battles on more than one occasion, and it was sickeningly terrifying. Danny couldn't shed his nature to size up Dad. Like jungle cats, they went nose to nose. Danny was a few inches taller than Dad. Instinctively, Dad crouched even lower and sidled closer to Danny's swelling chest and clenched fists. Danny's go-to action was to create space between them by raising his hands to shove Dad away, but Dad acted faster with a strategy in mind. As soon as Danny flinched, Dad's arms, like pit vipers, struck Danny's ears in rapid succession. After knocking him off balance, Dad leveraged for a stance to encase Danny in a chokehold or arm-bar. After ensnaring Danny, Dad held him there until he'd vented the greater portion of Danny's steam. Dad was fast and accurate. I believe he learned his moves from the professional wrestling matches he and Grandpa Stanger attended. At some point, we all tested Dad's authority, and it was never a win for either side.

#

Joe was a social butterfly and kept a collection of female friends at school and church. He carried himself with an elegant air and with equally matching clothes and sarcasm. Joe was unwittingly entertaining. He moved through a room as if he owned it and treated all that were present as serfs or peasants. He held his head high and swung his arms with the inner side of his wrists exposed as if under a royal benevolence or as a godly prince among mere mortals.

He liked to rile his ladies at church by publicly questioning their choice of outfit and whether it was appropriate for the season or in keeping with religious standards. If that didn't extract the response he was looking for, he brought their attendance or potential tardiness under review and even questioned their dedication to his friendship. He was relentless and continued his prodding until he elicited a squeal or a volley of similar attention. After pulling their trigger, he resounded with a laugh like the bray of a donkey, embraced them, and patted their backs as if he'd saved them from choking.

Once they realized that he had them, they giggled and struck at him with their headscarves saying, "Joey, I'm gonna' get you!"

He shared similar affections with everyone he encountered; it was his way of tearing down social barriers and softening people's fears. He could use this tool maliciously, too, but in defense of his boundaries.

Joe handled most of the housework and took it on himself to dress our home with decorations. He challenged Mom with ideas for wallpaper, paint schemes, carpeting choices, and window coverings. He pressed her to clothe the house in floral motifs but couldn't compete with Mom's love of Harvest Gold. Still, he gleefully accepted the consolation prize of painting his room a lovely shade of lavender and framing his single window with lace and gossamer. Once again, he left us males of the household rolling our eyes and shaking our heads. He wore our confusion like a badge of honor.

#

By the end of summer, Danny and Laura married. Danny's friends from Martinsville were part of the wedding party. It was good to see him with them again and listen to the accounts of their adventures. Danny looked slick in his gray-and-black tuxedo. Its cut accentuated his muscled armature. He usually walked off his toes, which gave a noticeable bounce to his step, but on this day, he seemed to float a few inches above the ground.

#

We were proud and excited by the prospects of our growing family. The addition of Ted, Laura, and the promise of Carrie's pregnancy permitted the final fibers associated with the loss of Garnna and Shelam to unravel and recede into what seemed like a fragment of an awful dream.

CHAPTER 4

The Road
(10 Years Old)

FRIDAY, SEPTEMBER 25, 1981, was Joe's eighteenth birth-day. He was a junior at Lapel High School. His acne was in full bloom, and the boys at school called him "Pizza Face" and "Fag." Those taunts didn't seem to bother him; Lamech and I branded him with crueler titles.

On that rainy afternoon, Joe rested his head against the school bus window. He looked tired but weaving your way through adolescence—especially as someone who doesn't fit the standard mold—drains you. As our conveyance edged up to the driveway, Joe snorted, brayed, and clapped his willowy hands. He grabbed his books, launched from his seat, and stood in the door well, rapping on the closure until the weary driver released him like a bird from a cage. As I moved up the aisle, I viewed what excited him. Carrie and Ted's car and a few others were in the driveway. Joe had an audience.

Joe rushed through the front door and into the dining room, where Carrie was changing the table cover. He was giddy with excitement. He rounded the corner into the kitchen to find Dad's brother and sister-in-law, Uncle Bill and Aunt Vera, who had driven from Texas for their annual pilgrimage to visit family and friends. Dad was home early, and Joe's friendly neighbors were arriving. He flitted around the house laughing and joking but kept a critical eye on the place settings and decorations Carrie was arranging. There was a substantial focus on Joe's birthday cake recipe Mom secured from a friend. Mom, Carrie, and Joe assembled the creamy ingredients for Next Best Thing to Robert Redford and laid them out in an aluminum pan.

As royalty, Joe presided over the gathering. He gushed with appreciation as he opened cards and gifts. He returned pokes and jokes with comedy and quips. As the evening wore down and our neighbors left for their homes, Uncle Bill asked Joe what he planned on doing after graduation. Joe responded that he was interested in going to floral design school and wanted to be a florist. This admission brought a few snide remarks from Ted and Lamech, but Uncle Bill silenced them with respect for Joe's intention to better himself. As the conversation waned, I segued from the table to the couch to watch the *Dukes of Hazzard* and fell asleep to the brassy intro to *Dallas*.

I awoke the next morning in an eerily quiet house. I rolled over on the couch to look toward the dining room and through blurred eyes, I recognized our neighbor, Mrs. Erwin, sitting in the rocking chair behind me. I suddenly realized I had kicked off my pants in the middle of the night and reached to cover myself, but I didn't have a blanket.

Exposed and embarrassed in my skivvies, I asked her, "Where's my mom?"

She replied, "She's at the hospital with Joe. She asked me to sit with you until she came home."

Confused, I asked, "Why are they at the hospital?"

With trepidation, she responded, "Joe got really sick last night, and they took him to the hospital by ambulance."

I searched, "Is everybody there?"

"No, your aunt and uncle went home a little while ago. I think it's just your mom and dad."

"Where's Lamech?"

"He's still in bed."

I tried to pretend I wasn't mostly naked as I pulled on my pants in front of Mrs. Erwin.

She asked, "Can I fix you something to eat?"

"No, I'm okay." I felt awkward, sitting alone with her. I left the room and went down the hall to solidify what she told me. Through Lamech's partially open door, I saw him sleeping. I continued to Joe's room, which was empty. A faint light came through the lace blinds and softened the harshness of scattered clothes, upended gift boxes, and bedsheets twisted, pulled to the floor. My bedroom and my parents' room were vacant.

While I tried to process what had happened while I was slumbering, I wedged my feet into my TRAX tennis shoes and slipped out of the garage's service door. A few steps into the lawn—thinking, I didn't want to be alone with Mrs. Erwin, and I didn't need a babysitter—I found the top half of a JC Penney clothing box filled with a creamy paste. It looked like Next Best Thing to Robert Redford. I wondered why someone had put the remains of the dessert in a box and left it outside. Within a few seconds, I realized it held vomit and was leaking into the grass. I figured it must be the contents of Joe's stomach. I remembered the cakes' consistency and fullness in my mouth and wished I hadn't eaten it. I turned my head away, squeezed through the chain-link gate, and walked around the neighborhood.

It was just after dawn; the roads and the yards were devoid of activity. Rain fell overnight, and there were traces of fog toward the swamp on the addition's backside. The rising sun cast the mist gold. Mr. Givens was in his shop, moving paint cans from one side to the other. Mr. Davis's garage door opened, and he backed his orange 1969 GTO onto his driveway. I did several laps around the subdivision and hoped for Whitey to come outside, but I knew it was too early. Eventually, I wandered home.

Mom returned, pale and shaking, and shared with Lamech and me the events of the night before and the current situation. After midnight, a rhythmic pounding emanating outside their room awakened Mom and Dad. Initially, they thought Uncle Bill was jokingly disturbing their sleep. This misconception lasted until they realized the sound came from Joe's room. Dad and Uncle Bill entered Joe's room and found him disfigured in a convulsive seizure. Uncle Bill called for an ambulance, and it transported Joe to St. John's Hospital in Anderson. By the time they arrived at the emergency room, Joe was listless and unresponsive. Within minutes, his left side contracted, drawing his head to his collarbone, his left wrist to his right shoulder, and his knee across his groin. Injected with phenytoin, Joe gradually relaxed. They admitted him to the ward and scheduled a CT scan on Monday morning. The doctor didn't want to speculate on what caused Joe's seizures, but my parents' instincts unpackaged their matrix of experiences. They acutely knew; a little over ten years had passed since Shelam exhibited the same physical manifestation. They also understood where this road might end. The situation horrified them.

I remember little from the rest of that day other than sitting on the front porch with Lamech, our heads cradled in our palms, while people came and went. I felt something, though, and it made me sick inside. It seemed as if the earth shook, opening a fissure, and a dark substance crept through the ground.

#

On September 28, the CT scan of Joe's brain revealed an enormous mass in his right frontal lobe. The scan exposed, within us, every abject fear and foul memory of Shelam's last winter.

They transferred Joe to Indiana University (IU) Medical Center in Indianapolis for further assessment. The IU staff believed surgery was necessary, and they scheduled the operation for October 7.

#

On September 29, high blood pressure forced Carrie into the hospital. Her condition required emergency action, and they induced her labor five weeks prematurely.

On the night of September 30, my parents' twenty-third wedding anniversary, Carrie gave birth to a son, Terry Nathaniel Ingram. I was as excited to be an uncle as Mom and Dad were to be grandparents.

On October 1, my father's forty-second birthday, the doctors released Joe from the hospital to see his nephew and attend Lapel's homecoming weekend. Worried over Joe's potential for seizures, we registered childlike fears:

"Can Joe hold Terry, or is there a chance he could drop him?"

"Do we need to sit with Joe in the band section or view him from a distance?"

"Should someone wait in the bathroom with Joe while he showers?"

Although slowed by phenobarbital and shaken by his situation, Joe refused to accommodate our concerns. He pressed his knees together to form a slender lap and laid Terry there to hold while he brushed Terry's brow with the pads of his thumbs. Joe ran into the crowd at the homecoming game, where his girlfriends formed a cordon around him. If he had gone limp, I don't think he would have had the chance to hit the ground. There wasn't an option to enter the bathroom with him; he slapped and batted anyone who attempted to invade his privacy.

Mom and Dad returned Joe to the hospital on Sunday evening. The week before, they had split their work shifts to make sure they could always tend Joe at the hospital. The only time they came home was to shower and change clothes. Mostly, Lamech and I were on our own.

Mom stocked the kitchen with toaster pastries, frozen pork fritters, and Lipton Cup-a-Soup. Without Mom, I used an alarm clock to wake myself for school and gave myself enough time to eat, watch a cartoon, and meet the bus as it came to the edge of the driveway. When I returned from school, I cooked my dinner, watched a few cartoons, faked my homework, and spent the remaining daylight hours with Whitey.

#

I was in fifth grade and not doing well. I expected to fail. I formatted my mind from my previous year in Mrs. Abner's fourth-grade class. She was a frustrated woman. I questioned her desire to form children's minds as she seemed better suited to working in a penitentiary or possibly as a drill sergeant. She had little patience for anyone in the room, and at some point, everyone received her scorn. She verbally abused us, and she rained down derision from the top of her vocal range. I struggled to comprehend the material and felt safer not to expose my ignorance to her name-calling and character assassination.

Under her tutelage, I crawled further inside myself and spent most of the classroom hours drawing pictures in my notebook. Now, after almost three weeks of lackadaisical study, I was on my way to receiving my first F in math.

#

On the eve of Joe's surgery, we all wore our finest clothes and visited him at Indiana University. He looked happy—I'm sure he was, with the attention he got—but you could feel sobriety from him.

Early the following morning, we reported to the hospital to see Joe off to the surgery ward but received word they rescheduled his appointment for the next Wednesday. The doctors released him, and he came home with us for another few days.

Wednesday, October 14, was like a clan reunion in the large waiting area at the IU Hospital entrance. Our entire family, with several aunts, uncles, and friends, were there to visit with Joe and wait through the expected hours of brain surgery. I passed the time by reading magazines and perusing the vending machines.

Joe was in surgery for over three hours. Eventually, the surgeon called Mom and Dad to a compact conference room where he gave them dire news; he couldn't remove the whole tumor, and its structure was that of a glioblastoma (GBM). The median survival rate of people with a GBM is rarely longer than four years, but Joe's vital signs were excellent throughout the surgery, and his faculties appeared to be healthy.

They transferred Joe to the intensive care unit, where we could check on him throughout the day. In the cafeteria, Mom and Dad gave us the doctor's prognosis, and it had the effect of dropping everyone's hearts into their stomachs. The same type of brain tumor consumed Shelam.

The removal of Joe's bandages revealed a twelve-inch row of stitches, in the shape of a waning crescent moon, on the front-right quarter of his shaved head. He appeared callow and frail in his fetal position. I felt sick and sad for him, and my eyes watered.

After eight days, they discharged Joe and he returned home. They adjusted his medications to prevent seizures and swelling. His condition restricted him from driving and sequestered him in the house for six weeks. Instead of radiation and chemotherapy, monthly CT scans monitored his tumor.

The restrictions imposed on Joe's social life and range of travel frustrated him. He adamantly opposed missing classes and not graduating with his class. Lapel High School offered a tutor, Mr. Jakob, who came to the house three evenings a week to help Joe make up his lost time. After several physical complications and a substantial amount of study, he returned to school at the end of the semester.

#

Over the previous autumn, my parents drifted away from the church near Shady Side Park. They struggled emotionally and financially. They couldn't help their current fears and tribulations, and the resurgence of memories of Shelam and Garnna were debilitating. Dumbfounded by their plight, they turned inward and questioned themselves.

On a February morning in 1982, something spurred Dad awake and compelled him to take Mom and Joe to Potter's Church in Martinsville. At the morning service, during a "movement of the Spirit," they experienced an outward release of emotion. Tears cascaded down my parents' faces, and they felt a peace within that they hadn't encountered since following David. While kneeling at the altar, they committed themselves to follow God and the ways of the Pentecostal Church. Brother Potter recommended a small parish in Anderson, Temple Mount, believing it suited my parents' spiritual and religious needs.

The ensuing week, Mom forced me to dig through my closet for my plastic Buster Brown dress shoes, polyester suit pants, and a plaid button-up shirt for a Sunday morning visit to the new church.

#

The pastor and his parishioners were very welcoming. The congregation was small but had recently purchased a piece of land and planned on building a larger facility with more exceptional amenities. Dedicated to his godly charge, the pastor brandished scripture as a sword in one hand and as a gift in the other. He was an excellent steward of his beliefs and strove to diversify his teachings, which kept his people interested. Membership required participation in multiple evening services and labor at the construction site. My parents fully embraced the church and encouraged us to do the same. Carrie and Ted also chose Temple Mount as their spiritual home.

#

Ensuring that parishioners received the Holy Ghost and were baptized in the name of Jesus was the church's foremost creed. Potter's Church and Shady Side Church professed this same keystone. They held these Holy Ghost sessions every Sunday night, but any Wednesday Bible study, Friday youth service, Revival, or camp meeting was also an acceptable time to receive the Spirit of the Lord.

The procedure started at the end of every sermon. A Hammond organ or a piano laid out soulful background music while the minister used scripture to caress everyone's mind, calling them to the altar. When anyone without the Holy Ghost stepped beyond the front pew toward the altar, those that had previously received the Holy Ghost gathered around them to lay hands on them and pray out loud, beseeching the Lord to save their souls.

The prospects raised their hands and prayed to God, sometimes for hours, their arms being held up by those around them. They wept, repented, pleaded, and offered promises. Their dialogue often slurred and trailed into unintelligible strings of discourse; this was called speaking in tongues and was considered evidence of God's spirit. A salty minister walked from candidate to candidate and pressed a trained ear close to their mouths, hoping to recognize an inflection or a memorized syllable that signified the Holy Ghost was present.

When the prayer attendants witnessed the Holy Ghost, they confirmed its presence to a minister by triumphantly pointing at the recipient while howling, "They've got it!"

With this information, the organist played in free form, increased the tempo, and swelled the worshippers' intensity. The music spurred old ladies into shouting and young men into dancing; moved by the Spirit, they performed a shuffling, flat-footed hop like I'd witnessed mountain people do on the TV show *Hee Haw*.

After their emotions were spent and the Holy Ghost stopped pouring out its spirit, the organist released the Hammond from intelligible songs and let the Leslie speaker whisper out breaths of quiet inspiration, which soothed the attendees' hearts. A few unfulfilled but earnest seekers of the Spirit swayed in the prayer warriors' embrace as the pastor walked to the pulpit and spoke words of encouragement. He offered to baptize anyone who sought to cleanse their souls and take on the name of Jesus Christ. If they accepted his offer, he stepped into an ancillary room to shed his suit coat for a pair of fishing waders while someone took the prospect to the basement to change their clothes for a white smock.

When both parties were ready, the pastor went down into the baptismal tank and called for the uninitiated. In the heated water, he explained to them the mechanics of being baptized and quoted scripture. He asked them to hold their nose while he expertly embraced them and prayed to the Lord. He recited the scriptural incantation for baptism and, on completion, fully submerged the sinner. Once he pulled the cleansed parishioner from the depths, the pastor proclaimed that Jesus had washed away all their sins and they were now a child of God. The announcement caused the organist to kick the Hammond into another round of thumping music, which spurred a joyful fervor of singing and dancing.

The outpouring of emotion and song swelled and collapsed like the waves in the baptismal tank until an attendant minister brought the congregation under control. With the restoration of order, he or she congratulated the reborn souls, relayed the schedule for the coming week, and closed the service in prayer.

#

Acceptance into the fold required one to follow a set of outward actions dictated by scripture:

> Judge in yourselves: is it comely that a woman pray unto God uncovered? Doth not nature itself teach you that if a man have long hair it is a shame unto him? But if a woman have

long hair, it is a glory to her: For her hair is given her for a covering. If any man seem to be contentious, we have no such custom, neither the churches of God. (1 Corinthians 11:13–16 KJV)

In like manner also, that women adorn themselves in modest apparel, with shamefacedness and sobriety; not with broided hair, or gold, or pearls, or costly array, but with good works. (1 Timothy 2:9–10 KJV)

Be not ye unequally yoked together with unbelievers: For what fellowship hath righteousness with unrighteousness? And what communion hath light with darkness? (2 Corinthians 6:14 KJV)

Love not the world, neither the things that are in the world. If any man love the world, the love of the Father is not in him. (1 John 2:15 KJV)

If any man defile the temple of God, him shall God destroy; for the temple of God is holy, which temple ye are. (1 Corinthians 3:17 KJV)

They distilled these verses into a list of rules to follow. The brunt fell on the women; the church barred them from cutting or coloring their hair, wearing jewelry, applying makeup, or sporting men's or tight-fitting attire, and the clothing they did wear had to fall below their elbows and knees. Everyone had a mutual cross to bear; to maintain membership, no smoking, drinking, cussing, listening to secular music, participating in worldly entertainment, or salaciously mixing with anyone not in the fold was permitted.

Your income was likewise subject to the church; it required a tenth of any financial gain as a donation. Time and monetary offerings were also necessary, enforced by scripture:

> Then there shall be a place which the Lord your God shall choose to cause his name to dwell there; thither shall ye bring all that I command you; your burnt offerings, and your sacrifices, your tithes, and the heave offering of your hand, and all your choice vows which ye vow unto the Lord. (Deuteronomy 12:11 KJV)

> Will a man rob God? Yet ye have robbed me. But ye say, "Wherein have we robbed thee?" In tithes and offerings. Ye are cursed with a curse: for ye have robbed me, even this whole nation. (Malachi 3:8–9 KJV)

#

The fight against the temporal—by Bible study—was a constant theme every Wednesday night. Self-proclaimed experts in satanism, the occult, and Bible prophecy were often guest speakers; the pastor gave them a three-night venue, with the Friday-night exhibition being the advertised cliffhanger. Slide projectors casting images of charts, graphs, photographs of current events, and artful photos of hell or demons prepared the ground for the main event. They mortared samples of suspect music, snippets of the newscast, and eerie sound bites of satanic voices into the voids to provide a solid foundation for the big show. The rhetorician expertly wove a verbal masterwork that had you either on the pew's edge or escaping to the restroom. The pastor expected every parishioner to bring a visitor with them, and most did. They needed folding chairs to seat everybody. The audience's density and anticipation of the final installment added substantial credence to the event.

Friday night started with the pastor leading a few uplifting songs. His sheep impressed him by filling the sanctuary with potential candidates for salvation. He welcomed the congregation and asked for an offering for the guest speaker. The ushers distributed brass plates and plastic buckets through the aisles to collect cash, coins, and checks. The pastor kept his comments short as he knew everyone was looking forward to the last presentation.

The guest speaker, with a grave demeanor, began his show with a prayer. The drama was rich and timed to perfection. He wielded a stream of dialogue like a veteran butcher opens a hog belly with a sharp knife. He called out demonic forces that battled for the souls of men. He sidestepped sensibilities and thrust questions of intent and dedication to Christ. He cued rock 'n' roll songs played in reverse; the dissonant and sinister-sounding enunciations and pictures of demonic possession chilled everyone to their core.

The audience was in quiet suspense as if expecting a violent thunderstorm. The evangelist left no stone unturned. Every modern or popular song was under his microscope. He informed us that all worldly music had a second and more perverse message. He sacrificed modern Christian music and continued down the line to encompass the black sheep of entertainment. Chubby Checker and his popularization of the twist was the very sexual nature of Satan. Jethro Tull channeled hell's sounds; the actual screams of the tormented were audible at specific volumes. He exposed KISS, secretly known as "Knights in Satan's Service," as a genuine evil. He illuminated the Beatles' practice of hiding messages in the song "Revolution 9." How could anyone know playing it backward revealed a request to be turned on by a dead man? "Turn me on, dead man." What did that even mean?

He laid out the list of artists, based on his reputable sources, that had certifiably sold their souls to Satan for fame and fortune. The only thing the Devil required, besides forfeiting your soul, was to lead the innocent youth to him like a modern-day pied piper. Led Zeppelin's *Stairway to Heaven* was a stairway to hell. The Eagles' *Hotel California* was a firsthand account of the ritualistic worship of Satan in the high desert of California.

It electrified the atmosphere as he continued to single out names and note actions and incidents of iniquitous behavior. He trailed out a list of musicians and bands such as Jimmy Page, Jerry Lee Lewis, Elvis Presley, Linda Ronstadt, Juice Newton, Dolly Parton, Styx, Foreigner, Rush, Judas Priest, Triumph, Journey, and Black Sabbath. With each name, he raised his voice and physical gestures. When he landed on Bob Seger, a vicious scream came from the darkened room. A sizable woman jumped from her seat, thrust both arms forward, pointed her fingers at him like daggers, and laid out a stream of cursing and profanity such as I'd never heard. It was as if a bomb detonated in the congregation's center, and it sent people gasping and ducking. For seconds, it dumbfounded the evangelist. Quickly, a pack of ushers and nearby ministers pounced on the lady and wrenched her, kicking and screaming, from the building. This action capped the show by providing material for the teacher's final rant about Satan, his demons, and their hatred for the enlightenment he'd spent the past hour sharing with us.

People quivered in their seats as he prayed in tongues and informed us that evil spirits were drifting through the congregation, intending to possess us should we not submit to Christ's protective powers. He opened the altar for prayer, and like a stampede of cattle, terrified souls broke and scrambled for the pulpit.

I remained where I was, wide-eyed and petrified. I looked to my left and my right at the vacant spots around me. Isolated, I closed my eyes out of fear, lest some rancorous spirit appear before me. The hair on the back of my neck stood on end in anticipation of clawed and twisted beings seeking to inhabit my skin. I prayed every fragment of incantation I could call to mind, from all the church services I'd ever attended, hoping to shield my vulnerable qualities from the Devil.

Like a statue, I held fast, trying to be as small and inconspicuous as I could. My eyes and hands remained clenched on the pew in front of me until I heard the pastor take the microphone and sing along with the organist as she played several gravely spiritual songs. The altar call continued with people crying and moaning. The pastor admonished everyone to repent of their sins and offer their souls to God. He solemnly commanded everyone to clean their homes of secular music and vice lest they fall under Satan's spirits of possession. That night, they baptized a few individuals and made appointments for those not ready.

When we arrived home from the service, Lamech and I cleared out our music collection, save a Beach Boys' *Endless Summer* album—not having been on the preacher's list—and deposited the stack of records in the garage. I wrapped myself in a sleeping bag on the floor of Lamech's room.

How could what I just went through be legitimate? I'd watched snippets of *The Amityville Horror*, *The Omen*, and *The Exorcist*; those were scary stories with terrifying images, but I figured they weren't real. Maybe they were true? I'd never witnessed so many adults—masons, meatcutters, bankers, salesmen, ministers, teachers, and doctors—invested so strongly in anything.

I dared not open my eyes when Lamech turned off the bedroom light. It terrified me knowing some haint, noticing my lack of commitment to God, could have followed me home and lurked in the corners, ready to attack me as soon as everyone slept. I'd read about dogs being able to smell fear, and I assumed that demons might have the same ability. If that were the case, I was an easy target. I did not understand how to deal with this new special warfare; the way I saw it, the Devil's henchmen might be working for God. I knew the end of the world would be tough, and now I had to worry about things I couldn't see. I fell asleep wondering how to avoid detection.

As the church harangued parishioners with fearful doctrine and orders to separate themselves from the world, I entrenched myself in isolation. I trusted no one. I couldn't count on any lasting relationship because I believed everyone was saved from calamity or compromised by iniquity. Although I loved my parents and my siblings, it didn't matter, as I didn't feel I was like them. I wished I could be around Unck to talk about my fears; I thought he might have a way to deal with this situation, but I knew a phone conversation wouldn't remedy my dilemma. I considered talking to Dad but quickly dropped the idea as he was the driving force that pushed us into Temple Mount. Carrie didn't seem like an avenue to address my concerns; she followed the instruction at Potter's Church, embraced this religion, and Ted, Terry, and their farm saddled her.

#

Schoolwork was a problem for me; I didn't understand compli-
cated math, and grammar was challenging as I failed to comprehend diagramming sentences. My memorization skills for
vocabulary and science were weak. Dad tried to aid me with
my homework, but it was fruitless. I didn't grasp his methods, and my ignorance frustrated him. He realized he couldn't
help me when his instruction reduced me to tears. I accepted
my limitations. To reduce any negative impact on my parents,
the only graded papers I brought home were the ones with
high marks. When I received Ds and Fs on my report cards,
I artfully changed them to Bs with the proper application of
erasers and colored pencils. Before returning the cards to my
teacher, I removed the changes I'd created, and no one was the
wiser. Fortunately, she did an expert job explaining percent-
ages and associated the concept with our schoolwork that comprised our six-week and semester grades. I could manage ratios
in my mind as I could visually associate them with coins and
measurements on rulers. At that point, I recognized I could let
facets of my responsibilities slide and focus on the high-value
items that determined a passing grade.

#

The weeknight projects at the church construction site drew
my parents' focus away from my schoolwork and momentar-
ily distracted them from their anxiety over Joe's condition and
medical bills. The vision the people of Temple Mount had was
akin to David's intentions with Padanaram. Mom and Dad
loved applying themselves to community efforts, especially
ones that were flourishing. They immersed themselves in the

work as they did with the Lapel Band Boosters, Lapel Lions Club, Boy Scouts of America, and every other civic activity vital to them. As soon as Dad got home from Universal Tool, Mom forced a hastily prepared meal down our throats, then we rushed to the construction site and busied ourselves with manual labor.

I enjoyed being around the churchmen and watching them work; it reminded me of being with Mr. Cooper. Seeing them in this environment, removed from the religious context, made them appear more human, and I could meet them on equal ground while I swept dirt, picked up scrap materials, and organized hardware.

Dad was quick to make friends. The group appreciated his industriousness, knowledge, experience, and humor. The churchmen addressed one another as "Brother," so they called my Dad "Brother George," and he became buddies with Brother Dave, Brother Darryl, Brother Charlie, Brother Ray, and Brother Richard.

That spring, Dad and his friends chartered a bus to attend the Indianapolis Boat, Sport, and Travel Show. They invited me, and the venture was reminiscent of my time with Unck and Mr. Cooper. I loved watching them banter back and forth. They noted each other's vice for particular species of fish. They chided Brother Charlie over his many secret fishing holes and how his retirement from labor would substantially decrease the overall fish population, if not drive it into extinction. They wondered out loud about Brother Dave's ability to fit or not fit his round body into a pair of fishing waders, and if he did fit, how he would get out of them.

They twisted Brother Dave until he stood up, pointed a finger, and stammered at them, "Y'all are fortunate Jesus reformed me from my sinful days! If not, I'd beat y'all like laundry on a rock and hang y'all all out to dry!" His response brought laughter from all of us.

#

Saturday, June 12, 1982, was sunny and warm. I was eleven. I'd just escaped the fifth grade and was feeling high on the freedom of summer. Joe's seizure and surgery seemed distant. The mental storm that the church churned up multiple times a week still challenged me. I continued to question the quandary of my name, but I'd honed my woods skills and knew every trail, creek, and forest from my house to the White River and the surrounding hamlets. World War III was on my horizon, but Uncle Bill sent me his old Army gear in the mail. Its fit on my shoulders comforted me. I squared away the magazine pouches with a survival kit and a few cans of C rations. I considered myself capable. I felt as spry as the tree frogs I heard calling at night from the neighborhood swamp.

That afternoon, I entered the house from the backyard as Dad and Danny came home from a day's toil at Universal Tool. They shed their boots at the front door, unbuttoned their shirts, and jokingly vied over who needed a shower the most. Dad laughed and swung his arm to cuff Danny's head. Danny sidestepped, missed Dad's reach, and slipped past him. Danny was moving toward the bathroom when a look of confusion took hold of his face. He stumbled, paused, and crumpled to the floor.

At the foot of the dining room table, struggling and twisting as if he were in the maw of a predator, he howled, "Jesus! Help me!"

Dad, Mom, and Laura rushed to his side. His cry for help made me shiver; I'd never witnessed Danny ask for help, let alone panic, in any situation. I made my way to him from behind the table. I felt cold with fear as I saw his eyes roll, exposing their veined whiteness. He choked with froth in his mouth and repeatedly slammed his head against the floor while a crippling grand mal seizure disfigured his legs, arms, and hands. Laura was crying and screaming Danny's name. Dad prayed out loud while trying to restrain him from injuring himself on the table and chair legs. Mom leaped for the phone to call an ambulance. I backed away in horror and felt my stomach churn as I watched my indomitable brother jerking uncontrollably on the floor.

In the emergency room, they scanned Danny's brain. Even though my parents offered the physician Shelam and Joe's medical history, he remained unmoved in his assessment of the CT results and his opinion that Danny had experienced an epileptic seizure. A few days later, they prescribed barbiturates for Danny and released him from the hospital.

The following week, in our dining room, we attempted to celebrate Danny's twentieth birthday. The celebrations felt half-hearted, if not heartless. Eight months had passed since Joe's seizure. Joe's condition improved and he regained his driving privileges, but Danny's seizure and its possible cause hung around everyone's neck like a millstone. Danny's olive skin had faded to gray and he was somber. The medications slowed his humor and slurred his speech. Watching him open presents while feigning joy was heartbreaking. When Danny cut into his chocolate cake, I had flashbacks to Joe's birthday and the morning after his seizure. I felt an icy dread inside. I wondered if I would have a fit of convulsions. A bitter taste rose in the back of my throat, and it was hard to breathe. I chewed on my piece of cake and chocolate ice cream but didn't register a flavor. I couldn't swallow.

I excused myself from the table and fled to Whitey's. I didn't want to think about Danny and Joe, the Bible, or my prospects of burning in hell. I wanted to be happy and have the fun that every other kid my age seemed to enjoy.

As I stared at my feet while walking to Whitey's, I tried to push the image of Danny contorted on the floor out of my mind. I scuffed my shoes on the pavement to stop the replay of his scream.

Why didn't he stop having a seizure after he cried out for Jesus to help him? That's what the pastor of the church said to do when confronted by trouble. He claimed the name of Jesus had power over everything; demons trembled in fear, and people were miraculously healed when they invoked Jesus's name. They had baptized Danny, and they said he got the Holy Ghost. Joe had gone to church since we lived in Martinsville; going to church was his paramount activity. Why was this happening to them? Were they doing something wrong, or maybe Jesus wasn't as powerful as the church thought he was?

I thought about the sock puppets from Potter's Church. I imagined the lifeless feel of the plastic head of Jesus stitched to an old sock and felt disgusted. Is that what the religion was, a crude toy that had no power but what a human hand gave it? The dialogue from the pulpit had me believing they knew how to keep people safe from harm; if a person fell in harm's way, they had a connection to God that would miraculously deliver them from evil.

My brothers were encountering evil. Garnna and Shelam, as babies, met evil and perished. Why? They couldn't have done anything wrong. My parents went to church while my sisters died. I'm sure they prayed for my sisters like I'd heard them pray for Danny and Joe. I'd prayed for my brothers; I didn't expect my prayers to have any impact, but I wanted them to get better.

I made it to the stoop of Whitey's house, knocked on the door, and let myself inside. I found him in his room working on stop-motion animation with an old 8mm camera. I didn't mention what had happened to Danny. I didn't want him asking questions or telling me he was sorry. The church had been showering my family and me with sympathy for our plight. Their offerings made me feel sour and resentful; I couldn't deduce why it made me feel that way, but it did. I didn't want to feel that from Whitey. I didn't want to talk about any of the subjects that worried me, and I didn't want him to treat me like something damaged or weak. If I were with Whitey, I could be a different person. I could laugh and create things. I could hide my guilt and fear of death and disease. Whitey and his family never questioned my feelings or asked about my life at home. To them, I was Sharek, Whitey's friend, who liked to build Tamiya models, draw pictures, collect comics, and listen to music. I didn't want them to know what was happening with me. They were an oasis, and I wanted to keep it that way.

#

Danny had more seizures. They came in clusters and were as wrecking as his first. Changes to his prescriptions halted his convulsions for weeks, but they always returned with a vengeance.

Mom and Dad pressed Joe's doctor to provide a second opinion on Danny's condition. He agreed to accept Danny as a patient and requested his CT scans for review, but weeks passed without a response. Mom, twisted by the unknown, called the practitioner and demanded his opinion on Danny's films.

The doctor stated, using words that tore through us like a blade through grass, "It looks like there is a brain tumor, but we'll need another scan in three months to be sure."

September was three months away. A date—ninety days in the future—was something I could ignore if not forget, but for Danny, the wait was agonizing. He worked at the tool shop every day, and seizures sapped him as often. He hoped the doctors were wrong, but he thought a remedy such as Joe's was his best option. The MRI scan bore down on him like an avalanche and he couldn't get out of its way. His temperament darkened and he was sullen. He didn't joke with me as he did before. He was quiet and his eyes were vacant. I was scared to ask him what was on his mind; I knew it was the same thing on everyone's mind and I didn't want to hear him say it aloud. I didn't want him to say he was afraid or worried about having a brain tumor. I didn't want to hear him admit he was sick. I also didn't want to, by chance, stir him to anger. He carried a rage just below his medicated surface, and it was unwieldy.

Worry and grief consumed Mom and Dad as they applied themselves to their daily tasks. They both worked as many overtime hours as they could to pay Joe's medical expenses and continued to maintain their commitment to the church. Lamech devoted the summer to working on Ted and Carrie's farm. Joe busied himself with the housekeeping while I mowed the lawn and weeded. As soon as I completed my chores, I tried to get as far away from the fear and dread as possible. I spent as much time as I could with Whitey. If he wasn't available, I went to my forest to see the beech tree and walk around the pond.

#

Later that summer, I joined little league football. My team was the Green Bay Packers. The coach lived in our addition and transported me to practice on the weekends. I played offensive and defensive end. My first game coincided with Danny's appointment for the MRI. I made my first touchdown during that game; I caught a twenty-five-yard pass spiraled to the end zone. Mom and Dad weren't there to witness it, and I didn't mention my accomplishment to anyone.

I enjoyed going to practice every day, right after school. It filled up the time when I usually struggled with homework. I was proud to carry my pads and helmet onto the bus every morning; next to drawing, it was the only thing that made me feel positive.

When I played football, I felt like I was doing something that would make Danny proud. Whitey and I and the other boys played ball games in the neighborhood, and I was okay. Playing on a proper field with real pads made me feel legitimate. I wanted to be like Danny. I wanted to be as fast and tough as he was. Since I first registered his presence in Martinsville, I wanted him. I wanted to be as close as I could to him. He was everything I felt I wasn't. He was powerful and didn't give a damn about anything. He made his own way and wasn't afraid of anyone or anything.

Danny's MRI confirmed he had a tumor; it was aggressive, lodged between his brain's two halves, and inoperable. I couldn't be proud of my sporting ability. Not now. I thought being good at something he once was might make him feel bad. Besides, no one in the family was very interested in sports.

My coach noticed my parents never came to my games. When driving to and from practice, he inquired about them, and I shrugged off his questions and stared out the window. I didn't want to describe what had happened with my family over the past year.

One Saturday evening, his curiosity got to him; he asked to meet my parents on the way home from practice. I led him into the dining room where everyone was sitting, having just finished dinner. He introduced himself, offered pleasantries, and asked Mom and Dad what they thought of my football prowess. They blinked at him and asked him what he meant.

He glanced at me and asked if I'd told them about my touch-downs and the points I'd scored.

They said, "No, he hasn't," while I stared at my cleats.

He put his arm around my shoulder and informed them I was fantastic and would make the All-Star team. His visit created an uncomfortable silence. Everyone looked at me with confusion in their eyes. Sensing the awkward environment, he broke the pause and excused himself from the house. Dad asked me why I hadn't told them about my success, but I couldn't explain. I could have slid under a rock without touching its bottom.

I played football until the end of the season. I made the All-Star team but sat on the bench more often than not.

#

Shortly before Christmas, Joe's biannual CT scan illuminated substantial tumor growth and his doctors immediately sched-uled surgery. Over the next five months, he underwent five more surgeries, stemming from infection in the palm-sized por-tion of bone that covered the nest of cancer in his brain. This withered everybody involved, and we sank within ourselves.

Holidays, birthdays, and normally momentous events couldn't cast a warm glow over us. Everyone but Lamech and I, with legitimate reason, pressed themselves to the church like soldiers to trees during an artillery barrage. Lamech withdrew from the assemblage, and I felt something festering inside me.

Over the past few years, I'd experienced a lot of fear. Beyond the threats of character flaws, hell, demonic possession, and the Apocalypse, I was not only afraid for my brothers but also for my physical wellbeing. The math of our situation bore on me—Garnna had died and Shelam, Joe, and Danny had brain tumors—and I didn't expect to escape the evident family plight. With every odd twitch of my eye and random headache, I suspected a tumor lay quietly tunneling inside my head. I believed it would expose itself in full glory with a seizure at school, on the playground, or at home alone while everyone else was at the hospital with Joe or Danny. I worried about pissing myself and choking on my tongue during a grand mal seizure. Daily, I wondered what region of my skull the doctors would have to remove. The mundane things concerned me, like how fast my hair could grow back and how long I'd be out of school. I tried to predict how slurred my speech would be and which of my classmates would make fun of me. At darker times, I thought of stealing Dad's gun from his top drawer and blowing out my brains instead of undergoing surgery.

Deep into winter, I felt something slip in my heart; all the fear rolled over like a ship in a storm, and I wasn't afraid anymore. It was similar to something I'd learned while standing in the cold, waiting on the bus; if I relaxed against the wind, it seemed to blow right through me, almost like I wasn't there at all. I let the fear blow through me. Instead of being cold and afraid, I felt nothing. At first, I thought this was a marvelous thing, and it was—letting everything through without thinking—until I encountered hate. The crux of this change took place as my well-intentioned sixth-grade teacher called me to stand beside his desk and face my classmates while he laid out my family's plight and asked them to pity me.

Pity—that's what it was. That's the feeling I hadn't been able to understand. Pity was the thing I'd felt from everyone that knew about us. The pity showered on me made me recoil and hide my feelings. That's what I didn't want Whitey or anyone else to feel for me. Pity, regret, and disappointment. I had my burden to carry, and it tore at me to have to shore up anyone in the vicinity that knew my story. I'd focused diligently on hiding my association with the church and was critically secretive about my family's weakness. I'd already imagined everybody could see my problems as if they were grime on my clothes. Now, exposed in front of my peers as the weak link in a chain or something that was a physical failure and worthless, I felt like trash, and it made me furious.

I didn't want the church. I didn't want my family. Most of all, I didn't want an unable god to do a damn thing. Fuck it all. Fuck it all, and let come what will.

I quit trying to make friends and be friendly. I accepted the fact I was a prisoner and, with that, I looked for an escape. I pined to get away, and I did. I went with Whitey, kept my mouth shut about Joe and Danny, and didn't give a damn.

CHAPTER 5

Little Light
1983–1985 (11–14 Years Old)

IN THE SPRING of 1983, I was eleven years old. Joe graduated from high school; it was a monumental accomplishment. He bore the surgeries and maintained his schoolwork with grit and determination. He eventually regained his driving privileges, which brought him great joy as he would attend floral design school in Indianapolis. It was good to see him doing well, and it seemed to lighten everyone, including Danny.

#

I should have moved in with Whitey; I was at his house more than my own, and we were always together. If there was anything fun to do, we did it, and our activities were relatively wholesome until one Friday night after his parents retired for the evening. As soon as they ascended the stairs, Whitey pushed away from the kitchen table, where we were drawing copies of Frazetta posters, and disappeared down the hall to the bathroom. A few minutes later, he returned with a gallon jug of vodka. I stared at him, wide-eyed, as he tucked his chin and let a half smile curl the corners of his mouth. With a devilish pride, Whitey poured two old-fashioned glasses full of the clear liquid. He asked me to get the orange juice out of the fridge and divide us two similar-sized quantities. I agreed and placed my work next to him. He picked up both glasses of booze, handed me one, and asked if I was ready.

I asked him why we needed the orange juice, and he pontificated, "They call this a Screwdriver. We knock back this vodka and chase it with the juice to wash the taste out of our mouths." He wryly winked at me and downed his glass of vodka as fast as he could. I followed suit, and we both fumbled for the chasers.

Whitey shook his head, wiped his mouth, and declared, "That's pretty good!"

I couldn't agree with him, but we poured another batch, topped off the jug of liquor with water, and Whitey returned it to the cabinet below the bathroom sink. The next set of Screwdrivers was as bad as the first, but the deed was empowering.

To continue our devilry, we took in some night air by slipping out the house's back door. We wandered around the neighborhood, weaving and stumbling, and surrendered to buffoonery. Our entertainment reached a crescendo as, from the street, we spied a single illuminated square among the assemblage of darkened homes. Not forty feet from us, framed by the lace drapes of an open window, a lovely young woman was undressing in the amber glow of lamplight. Whitey and I glanced at one another, awestruck by eroticism, and stepped a little further into the shadows before returning our gaze to the most brilliant exhibit we'd ever seen. Fully exposed, she was breathtaking. Though excited, I felt guilty. I thought I was invading her privacy.

I mentioned my concern to Whitey, and he slapped the back of my neck and whispered, "Dummy, she's the one that left her blinds open!"

We continued to take in the view as she slowly turned to study her backside in a large round mirror. She ran her palms down her breasts and belly, across the tops of her thighs, settled them along the sides of full hips, and rotated in profile. She repeated this procedure more than a few times. Eventually, she confirmed an assessment and crossed the room to extinguish the light.

Whitey and I looked at one another, breathless, and whispered in unison, "Jesus Christ!"

The next morning, I woke, not remembering having gone to sleep, and crept out of Whitey's house. My head was pounding and I felt sick. I staggered home, not knowing what was wrong with me, thinking I'd sleep the rest of the day. On my arrival, Dad notified me we were all going to church.

I asked why, and he said, "We, as a family, have all volunteered to clean the church before service on Sunday." I questioned the day, believing it was Saturday. Dad confirmed that it was Saturday and that he wanted to make sure we were ahead of schedule. We left for the church in due order, and my confinement in the back seat with Lamech and Joe compounded my illness.

We pulled into the gravel parking lot and walked into the building. Beforehand, Lamech and I affirmed with one another that this was a stupid idea. Just inside the church, Lamech, like a colt under a saddle, bucked at Dad's instruction. Dad—never one to tolerate disrespect—quickly grabbed Lamech by the arm and kicked him in the ass three or four times. After witnessing that bit of measured discipline, I immediately opted to find anything nearby that needed a thorough cleaning. Although I felt as if someone had run me over with a car and didn't like where I was or what I was doing, the vision of the woman in the window made it all more bearable.

#

Mamaw's health declined. By the end of June, we moved her from Martinsville to live with us. I surrendered my bedroom to her and transferred my bed into Lamech's. He wasn't happy with the situation but didn't have an alternative.

Mamaw didn't seem the same. She'd lost her proclivity to look in my eyes and talk with me like a peer. She didn't ask for my help anymore, and I was too large to lie across her lap. She slept in Dad's recliner most of the day and into the evening. Her snoring drowned out the audio from the TV, but we didn't mind. Mom spurred her to converse over dinners, but Mamaw didn't have much to say other than to comment on the quality of the food and state she was sorry she was so tired. She often excused herself from dinner before we finished, and with the aid of her aluminum walker, carefully traveled down the hall to sit in her bedroom. Before everyone headed to sleep, she'd emerge in a cotton nightgown and make her way to the bath. Her hair, released from the bun at the rear of her scalp, was like spun silver and draped to the small of her back. The scene evoked a memory of lying under quilts on her davenport and watching the same beautiful spectacle. I remembered her asking me if I'd like to move from where I was to sleep in her room on Papaw's bed, and her warning about the cold in there. I remembered lying with Papaw's comforter tucked under my arms, playing with my breath in the air, as she knelt to pray at her bed across the room. I recalled wondering how and why she trapped her incredible mane at the nape of her smooth neck. Now, I felt pain for her; I knew she didn't want to leave her home, and I could see her resignation at not having her own place to maintain or her precious mementos to keep. All she had to do was sleep.

#

Shortly after my twelfth birthday, Dad drove me up to Hartford City and dropped me off at a Pentecostal church camp. I was sullen and angry at my fate of being forced to spend nine full days—two hundred and sixteen hours—at church. I'd told Whitey where I was going, and he responded with a look like I'd punched him in the forehead.

A weed-filled pond, fed by an algae-choked creek, bisected the gravel campground. On the rise at the property's primary side was a metal tabernacle—the heart of the complex—where they conducted daily activities and nightly services. Nests of camper trailers and cinder-block latrines peppered the periphery of the estate. There was an air-conditioned chapel the church deemed off-limits; they considered it incompatible with a traditional camp meeting experience. The cafeteria was air-conditioned, but they reserved it for the elderly and infirm. The only other refrigerated space was a two-story concrete bunker that served as the girls' dormitory. Women, clothed in full denim jumpers, jealously protected the fortification. Like guard dogs, the chaperones patrolled the perimeter to call out boys who strayed too close to the entrance. There were other roving patrols—staffed by young adults—dedicated to the cause of limiting any serious adventure.

Lodging for the males was a cluster of cabins tucked in a wooded corner directly opposite—across the lake—from the girls' stronghold. My residence for the week was one of the musty shacks. I shared the hovel with four other boys from Temple Mount. Three of them were the Riggs brothers, and the fourth was Jerry Hilderbrandt. Jerry was a few years older than me and was, by the church's assessment, incorrigible. He refused to follow the religious standards of dress and openly listened to rock 'n' roll music. His mother—the driving force—pressed him into the church as his father was elderly and had no proclivity to steer Jerry to the altar.

Jerry cultivated himself a well-tailored image. His hair, always perfectly spiked on top, ended in a coiffed mullet. He pressed his shirts, and the collars stood to touch the earring that dangled from his left ear. His jeans, tightly pegged into his dazzling white Reeboks, invariably appeared to be new. Jerry never exerted himself and retreated to the rear of a building or a vehicle's back seat. Being feckless, the other boys and I put him on a pedestal as something we wanted to be. I'm not sure why he was at church camp—he had permission to disregard everything about it—but he was.

#

There was the opportunity to participate in wholesome activities such as singing in the youth choir, playing basketball, making crafts out of macaroni and popsicle sticks, or navigating a rowboat through the carpet of vegetation that was the lake surface. But all those endeavors exacted a toll in sweat and discomfort.

Every four hours, there was some mandatory gathering in the tabernacle. Although there were multiple wide openings in its sides, there was no air movement within its confines. Aqua Net–armored hair and antiperspirant were no match for the heat and humidity that came with being packed in there beside two hundred feverish bodies. Perspiration beaded on foreheads, wet the backs of necks, rolled down the insides of arms, and saturated clothing. The only highlight of the sweltering atmosphere was that it exposed brassieres through white blouses and caused the girls' cotton jumpers to cling and reveal their more exceptional shapes.

I quickly gained the impression that they built a traditional camp meeting experience on the foundation of having as many church services and Bible studies as possible while dampening sexual entertainment in a sultry environment.

\#

The godly duties did little to sway the principal purpose of every boy and girl, that being, to find a mate and wander off after the nightly services. The Riggs brothers and I, along with most of the other boys, hung out on the bridge over the creek. We searched the windows of the girls' bunker for signs of life. Our quarry was challenging; after each mandatory gathering, the girls beat a hasty retreat to their air-conditioned compound and remained there until the guard dogs pushed them out for the next tabernacle meeting. We goaded one another to press the cordon of denim-clad sentries and hail any female near the entrance. We hoped to signal a pliable resource into delivering messages of interest in dating. It took a fair amount of courage to stand exposed on the sunbaked gravel in front of the structure and proclaim your desire before all the darkened windows. To protect our pride, we occasionally sent a younger boy—as an emissary—who had no stake in the game.

\#

On Tuesday, just after breakfast in the cafeteria, I received notice from a female emissary—irritated by her mission—that one of her compatriots was keen on going out with me after the evening service. With a hand on her hip, she cocked her thumb over her shoulder and motioned at a covey of middle-school girls in the shade of an oak tree. She told me that the black-haired girl liked me and wanted to meet me. After I nodded and said I was interested, she pulled a folded piece of notebook paper from her purse and jammed it in my hand. With her task completed, she turned on her heels in the gravel and stomped off toward the girls' bunker.

I unfolded the note to reveal a fat cursive script that proclaimed I was cute. The assessment ended with two exclamation points. The following line was an instruction to meet on a bench near the rear of the tabernacle. The author signed off with a bubbly shaped autograph, "Sherry," and added a heart for emphasis.

I looked up from the note and waved at Sherry. As I moved in her direction, she broke from her group and made her way up the slope to the tabernacle's rear side. She disappeared around its corner, and by the time I rounded it, she was sitting on a bench. After an introduction, we acquainted ourselves with each other's backgrounds. She was from Kokomo and was part of a small Pentecostal congregation on its northern reach. She was a year older than me and was as interested as I was in going to church. She was pretty, so much so that it surprised me that she had an interest in me. We spent the rest of the day—between services—meeting at unobserved benches across the compound. We coordinated our seating inside the tabernacle to see one another, and eventually sat next to each other during the youth choir practice. The outside of her thigh was hot and firm against mine. Our arms touched, and we interlocked pinkie fingers without being noticed by the guard dogs.

Outside of learning about each other's schools and churches and dissecting the points of church camp we didn't like, we didn't say much. Nightly, we made up for our lack of discourse by sneaking off behind the air-conditioned sanctuary to make out. It surprised us to find that we weren't alone in our secret excursions. The woods on the north side of the chapel were devoid of light but filled with other couples engaged in the same activity. The roving patrols—mighty throughout the day—must have feared the dark.

#

On Thursday night, after walking Sherry to the bridge, I returned to the cabin just before curfew. Two of the younger Riggs brothers had been in the hut for a while and were throwing small objects into the window fan to see how far it would spit them back across the room. Jerry and the elder Riggs brother sneaked in a few minutes later. They'd had dates, and we talked about the evening. Jerry grew annoyed with the boys' antics, filled his hand with a pile of shaving cream, and flipped it into the fan, plastering the two Riggs boys. Jerry's action turned into a frolic, leaving the contents of his can of Brill deposited on the walls around the space.

The following day, the mother of the Riggs brothers stopped by the cabin to check on her boys and discovered the messy scene. In short order, we were all summoned to the shack by the elders of our church. When I arrived, they were helping old Brother Hilderbrandt up the steps. On entering, I experienced a full inquisition of how and why the property was so disrespectfully maintained.

Jerry was the focus of the insinuations and assumptions. He pleaded his case, implicating no one, and tried to defuse the situation by showing how easily he could clean the cabin with a damp towel. Brother Hilderbrandt—who couldn't see a fly on the end of his nose if he tried—had the scene explained to him as if it were a crime. Jerry's shoulders sank when his dad asked him why he'd done such a horrible thing.

At that point, the only thing Jerry could say was, "I'm sorry, Dad."

It was a disgusting display of overcorrection; they could have left old Brother Hilderbrandt out of the action, and Jerry wasn't any more responsible for the mess—if there was any—than the rest of us. I felt terrible for him; he didn't want to disappoint his father, and he tried to protect us from punishment. It didn't matter, though. After we cleaned up the cabin under the elders' supervision, they sent Jerry home with his father and removed the Riggs brothers to stay with their mother in a camper trailer.

Later that afternoon, Mom and Dad arrived for the evening camp meeting service, and the elders informed them of the crime. Dad walked me back to the cabin to verify that it was in good order. He didn't seem upset, but he admonished me to keep my nose clean. I spent the remaining nights in the hut by myself.

Sherry and I continued our daily schedule and our nightly escapes. It was sweet and exciting. On the Sunday afternoon before she returned to Kokomo, we exchanged addresses and promised to write—and we did—until the autumn when school started.

#

When I returned from church camp, Whitey was on vacation with his family. Being bored and not wanting to be inside the house, I took the 760 and an old model car out in the front yard. I placed the toy against the trunk of a pine tree and sat back against a maple and engaged myself in punching holes through its plastic hull. After eight or ten shots, the target was a disfigured carcass and no longer offered a challenge. Across the street, high in another pine, I spied the shape of a bird and aimed. The bird's silhouette was minuscule; it wasn't half as wide as the sight post. I squeezed the trigger and felt the rifle recoil.

In an instant, the bird rose from its branch in a flutter and tumbled through the tree. I couldn't believe I'd hit the mark at such a distance and knocked it to the ground. I'd thumped birds with the old Daisy BB gun, but they always flew away. I laid down the Crossman, pushed myself off the ground, and brushed the dirt off my jeans. I kept my eye on the place where the bird fell and saw no movement. Although alone, I felt observed from every angle. I walked to the road and stood there for a minute, trying not to expose the attention I was giving my last target. I realized I was short of breath; darting across the street, I pressed myself through the stand of pines.

I looked for the bird—wishing I wouldn't find it—but not twelve feet from me, I spied a gray lump on a footing of orange pine needles. I crawled on my hands and knees, pushing aside branches with my head until I came to the result of my action. The fowl I'd knocked from its perch was a mourning dove. It was upright with a wing outstretched. It tucked its head between its shoulders, opened its beak, and panted. I reached forward and pushed it with the backside of my hand, hoping it would fly elsewhere. It struck its other wing to the ground and rolled a few inches. I grasped it, folded its wings along its sides, and pulled it to my chest. I hoped I'd just thumped it silly, but that thought washed away with regret and shame when I saw beads of blood escaping through its smooth buff feathers. It craned its neck, struggling to get out of my palms, as its life pooled on its back and stained my thumbs. The dove surged and slipped a wing between my fingers, spattering my wrist with droplets of crimson. It squirmed a few more times and went limp. The dove's head lay on its side against my index finger with the light from above reflected on its glassy, coal-colored eye.

I felt sick and was angry with myself. I didn't want to kill it, but I did. I remembered watching mourning doves with Mamaw on her front porch and calling them to her yard because they were so special to her. I'd never been this close to one, and for the first time, I noticed how beautiful they were. I laid its body against the trunk of the tree and covered it with pine needles. I tried to wipe the blood from my hands, but it remained. I crawled out from under the trees and skulked home. I grabbed the gun and put it back in the garage locker. I believed I owed Mamaw and the world something I couldn't return.

#

In late September, Mom and Dad celebrated their twenty-fifth wedding anniversary by hosting a celebration and ceremony. Carrie and Joe decorated the house, and Mom hired a professional photographer to capture the event. On the front lawn, my parents repeated their vows in front of a large gathering of family and friends. Two days later, Mom took Mamaw to visit a geriatric physician. He immediately admitted Mamaw to the hospital.

Further tests confirmed advanced cardiovascular disease and failing kidneys. A CT scan of her chest exposed a rare defect, dextrocardia; she was right-hearted from birth. Mom, simplifying the terminology, told us that Mamaw's heart was backward. I didn't like how Mom labeled Mamaw's heart; the original description was accurate, Mamaw's heart had always been in the right place.

Two weeks later, while I was at school, Mamaw went to sleep and never woke up. The visitation and funeral of Dozy Garnet Stanger were in Martinsville. They held her in state at Potter's Church. Mom's brother, Uncle William, sang old gospel songs. His deep baritone voice was vibrant and passionate. Under Uncle William's woe, I couldn't stop the tears from filling my eyes. Big sobs rolled out of me when I witnessed Mamaw's elderly friends—dabbing their eyes and noses with embroidered handkerchiefs—as they passed her casket, spoke to her body, and kissed her brow. I knew a door had closed on something magnificent.

#

I missed a few days of school, and no one noticed but Whitey. He asked where I'd been, and it shocked him when I said Mamaw died. He questioned why I didn't tell him, but I didn't want to explain why. I think I hurt his feelings when I shrugged my shoulders and looked away. It must have bothered him enough to relay this information to his parents. A few days later, as I passed them in their living room, they stopped me and asked about Mamaw's passing. It scared me to divulge my grief; I felt if I did, I'd have to talk about all the other incidents raining down at home. Doing so would muddy the peace I enjoyed with Whitey's family.

I tried to brush over my feelings as quickly as possible without betraying what I was hiding, and blurted out, "Yeah, she died. That happens."

They immediately sensed something was wrong and paused before offering their condolences. I could see that my response was a mistake and made a mental note to not panic like that in front of anyone again. I thanked them and eased out of the room.

#

November blew in on the wind, and it was cold. Toll's flower shop hired Joe when he graduated from a floral design school. Mom and Dad bought him an old black Buick, and he was happily mobile. He'd had his semiannual CT scan; it showed recent tumor growth but not enough to merit another surgery. Danny continued to wade through weekly bouts with seizures and, characteristically, he dealt with them as he did with other aggressors. He was a scrapper and seemed indomitable. Lamech had paired up with a girl, Tonya, from church and spent as much time with her as possible. He purchased a 1966 Chevelle that was primed black. For Christmas, Mom and Dad gifted him a set of chrome Cragar wheels with new tires. Like all the accoutrements he'd owned over the years, the Chevelle was beautiful. Carrie was pregnant again, and everyone held it as a promise of light in the dark of Danny and Joe's struggles and Mamaw's passing.

#

January, frozen and full of snow, wasn't as bitterly cold as the twenty-second of February when the placenta in Carrie's womb separated and severed her unborn son, Ted Nicholas, from life. He was almost full-term, and it was shocking to see a lifeless baby.

Carrie lost a lot of blood and still in the hospital when we buried Ted. The wind ripped through the cemetery and drove what leaves remained from the autumn across the crust of ice and pinned them against gravestones as if they were being held accountable for trying to escape the winter.

Shadows

In March, I had headaches. They hit while I was at school, and by the time I got home, I couldn't do anything but lie on the couch and press my head into the armrest until I fell asleep. I often slept through dinner and into the next morning. My condition worried Mom and Dad, and they scheduled a CT scan for me. I preferred a headache over waiting for the results of the imaging. The report came back clear, but it didn't stop the problem.

If not wiped out from the pain, nightmares disturbed me. The dreams were repetitive in imagery and schedule. The visions consistently played out the scenario of submersion in the sea at night, sinking in a rusted cage, severed from its link to the surface. Outside the bars, prehistoric leviathans ground their armored mouths against the rotting iron of the enclosure. As I sank in the deep, I knew the crumpled hull's security was as deadly as escaping. I'd wake, out of breath, with my heart pounding in my ears. I'd lie there, trying not to sleep until my alarm signaled it was time to get ready for school.

#

Spring gave way to a sweltering summer. Our home wasn't air-conditioned, and the heat was unbearable at night. I'd lie awake with beads of sweat rolling down my temples while wishing for some breeze to move through the open window. On a Monday—just past midnight—I shoved the screen open, hoping to let some cooler air into my room. I leaned against the frame with my head outside and listened to crickets. I was scanning the street for anything of interest when I noticed silhouettes bounding from shadow to shadow like soldiers on an enemy objective. They were making their way along the road when they halted, concealing themselves in the pines next to my driveway. A shadow left the thicket and crept up the sidewalk to the bushes near the garage door. A pebble hit the glass—inches above my face—and about the same time, the shadow whispered my name and revealed its identity as Whitey. He closed the last twenty feet to the house and motioned for me to join him. I pulled on a pair of jeans and dropped my shoes and a shirt out the hatch. I squeezed through the lower sash opening, grabbed my kit, and slinked off with Whitey toward the pine trees. In the shadows, I could smell the booze on Whitey's breath. He was there with a few other knuckleheads from the neighborhood. He'd spent the previous hour rounding them up as he had me.

After I jammed my shoes on, we dodged the streetlights—slapping each other's shoulders as a signal to move—and made our way to the shadow behind the community church sign. Sitting with our backs against the brick wall, we chuckled at our current fortune and toked on half-smoked cigarette butts that Whitey had pilfered from his mom's ashtray.

I felt a great delight, lounging in the damp grass, shielded from the churchyard's spotlight. I felt like I belonged there, stealing the night with a close friend and a few shady compatriots.

We played several rounds of "Truth or Dare." The dares were relatively simple and mainly involved two options: pulling your pants down in the middle of the road under the streetlight or holding a breath of smoke as long as you could. The truth was a little more challenging; it was most likely riddled with falsifications or wasn't prized as uncommon knowledge.

We also held answers to questions of sexual accomplishments in disbelief, but "doing it" with the same handful of girls from school interested everyone.

Eventually, we burned through Whitey's fistful of cigarette butts and lay sprawled on our backs in the dew, making comments about the stars and profound ideas like alien contact and having sex with Whitey's sister's friends. We noticed that the crickets had quieted, and we figured it wasn't long before first light. We had no context of time as no one had a watch, so we agreed to split up and head back to our homes. Before wandering off, we committed to meet in the shadow of the church sign, just past midnight, every following night.

Emboldened by the darkness and stillness, we kept our nocturnal agreement. There was a sense of freedom, knowing the rest of humanity was sound asleep; without their presence, we felt we owned the night and all it shrouded. There were no yards we couldn't trespass, cars we couldn't touch, or activities that would bring reproach.

#

Throughout each sweltering day, we noted which homes had swimming pools and waited for the owners to go on their midsummer vacations. At night, like cat burglars, we scaled the fences of the vacated properties and swam naked in human-made lagoons without the slightest splash or disturbance that might wake a neighbor.

Whitey's sister Rose became aware of our escapades but kept our secret. With one of her friends, she followed us one night. They lagged a few yards behind and tauntingly cooed at us. Rose called to Whitey and said they wanted to go swimming. Whitey protested, and she threatened to expose our activities. Whitey countered with his knowledge of Rose and her associates getting into their parents' booze. His argument was weak; we'd been hitting the stash for almost a year. After a brief standoff, we led them to the nearest unoccupied estate and made our way over the fence. We boys opted to enter the pool with our shorts on, but to our delight, Rose and her friend pulled off their clothes and slipped into the tank. Justifiably so, the ladies commanded the center of the pool—rolling on their backs like mermaids in the moonlight—as we clung to the edges in juvenile amazement.

#

Later that summer, Dad conveyed me up to the Hartford City church camp. This time, I was looking forward to being there. Although I hadn't communicated with Sherry since the previous autumn, I hoped to rekindle what we had during our last camp meeting.

After depositing my bag in the cabin, I walked with the Riggs brothers out to the bridge to view the ladies occupying the bunker. I found boys from the Kokomo church and inquired about Sherry. I felt hurt for her when they told me she was pregnant and had dropped out of school.

The revelation about Sherry's state took the wind out of my sails. I mostly avoided the tabernacle and hid out in the hut until the evening services when Mom and Dad were in attendance. I went to the bridge a few times with notions of finding a date but ended up walking around by myself. I felt trapped, preoccupied with thoughts of the delinquent activities happening in the neighborhood.

#

After a summer of shenanigans, I entered eighth grade feeling wizened to the ways of the world. I held my head slightly higher and wasn't so worried about my classmates' opinions about me. Also, I discovered how to grease the social skids by applying bits of comedy that Whitey and I had honed. I felt a little comfort being in my skin.

#

Just before winter, Lamech traded his Chevelle for a late 1970s Camaro. He graduated from high school in January with plans to attend Purdue University in the autumn. To fill his time, he went to work with Dad at Universal Tool.

In late winter, Lamech acted noticeably different. He'd always been standoffish, if not sullen, but now he was mostly angry and easy to set off into a tantrum. He'd been busting his curfew every weekend and clashed with Dad regularly.

On a February night, after church, he was preparing to drive Tonya to her home in Alexandria when Dad forced him to take me along. There was a steady rain with a dense fog licking at the piles of snow on the roadside. Lamech was angry and driving faster than he should have. Something upset Tonya, but I couldn't discern what. She reached for the stereo, adjusted the speakers for the back seat, and cranked up the volume to a deafening level. There was no way I could hear what they were saying from my position in the back seat, but it appeared to be a vicious argument.

Lamech careened into Alexandria, spinning the steering wheel with one hand and showing no concern about hitting slush-filled craters along the road. By her actions, Tonya seemed to plead with him, but he remained as unresponsive as a stone wall. Lamech blew by her house and took haphazard turns through her neighborhood. He'd occasionally turn his head to her and force out words I couldn't hear. After an hour of racing through side streets and alleys, we skidded into Tonya's driveway. She leaned across the console toward him, grabbed his jaw, and forced him to face her. She spoke a few words to him, shut off the stereo, turned, and asked if I wanted her seat. She got out of the car and went inside as I moved to the front.

Lamech backed out of the driveway and rocketed out of town toward Anderson. I asked him if he was okay but he didn't respond. I tried to draw him out by commenting on the fog, but he turned the stereo up so loud I couldn't hear myself speak. A few weeks later, after a fight with Dad, he gathered his possessions and moved in with Tonya and her family.

In March, at a Wednesday-night Bible study, the pastor called Lamech and Tonya to the front of the church. He asked them to come and stand next to the podium as he stepped out from behind it. He stood between them and declared to the congregation that he wanted to quell any gossip that might wag people's tongues. Lamech and Tonya lowered their heads as tears rolled down Tonya's cheeks. He spoke about the trouble that young people could find for themselves. The pastor shared with everyone that Lamech and Tonya had committed grievous sins and were expecting a child. He stated that he expected them to marry as soon as possible. After leveling a full load of guilt at them, he released them from the pulpit and closed the service with a song. Tonya wiped her eyes as she walked down the aisle between staring parishioners. She escaped the sanctuary and fled to the restroom at the end of the service. Lamech returned to our family pew, chewed on the inside of his lower lip, and stared at the floor.

This revelation shocked me. I ached inside for Lamech and Tonya. I considered the things they talked about doing after high school and couldn't imagine how this would affect their plans. I looked along the pew at my other family members and saw tears in Mom's eyes, and Dad didn't seem far behind. I thought the announcement of conception should have been a glorious event, but this seemed as far away from that as anything could be.

Tonya dropped out of high school in April and married Lamech in May. Instead of accepting his scholarship in agriculture at Purdue, he opted to dig for a paycheck at Universal Tool and leased a residence in Alexandria. They were struggling with all the things a teenage family faces, and they fought a lot. A few times, I stayed with them at their apartment. Tonya and I spent the days around town doing what we could afford. In the evenings, Lamech rented videos on his way home from work, and we all looked forward to a fun night, but it always devolved into slamming doors and yelling at one another. I'd sit on the couch and try to ignore the fight boiling over eight feet away in the kitchen.

CHAPTER 6

Backwater
1985–1989 (14–17 Years Old)

BY NOVEMBER 1985, Laura, Tonya, and Carrie had each given birth to girls, and it was a heartwarming distraction from the disease evident in Joe and Danny. That winter, Joe's biannual CT scan revealed tumor growth that required another surgery and several months of radiation treatment. The treatments were so intense, the surgical site refused to knit and the forward half of his hair never returned to his scalp. Joe underwent a multitude of unsuccessful plastic surgeries to repair the damage from the radiation. Being permanently disfigured bothered him. Every time he went under the knife, he came out the other side a little darker in spirit. In the company of friends, he was strong, if not overbearing. Alone, he was coarse and easy to anger.

#

In the waning weeks of 1985, Lamech's financial state wrought him. He enlisted in the Army and shipped to Fort Sill, Oklahoma, while Tonya and their daughter moved in with us on Lone Oak Road. After Lamech completed Basic and Advanced Individual Training, he received orders to report to Germany for his first station assignment. As a lower-ranking soldier, he wasn't authorized to bring dependents with him. Anxiety rippled through the house; being geographically separated from a family member wasn't something anyone wanted. The consolation from Lamech's absence was the pleasure of having Tonya and my niece with us for an extended stay.

#

By now, I was a freshman in high school. I struggled with my studies as much as I did at being the type of son everyone thought I should be. After Lamech and Tonya's "grievous sins," Temple Mount knuckled down on its shepherding of youth. They instituted a mandatory Friday-night service for anyone under eighteen and required the parents to be there. Joe was in and out of IU Hospital every week. I didn't see much of Mom and Dad except on the weekends when we were at church or in a hospital waiting room. I was losing my time with Whitey, and when we got together, I'd drink until I passed out. Whitey's family sold their house and moved into another housing addition further north on Lone Oak. He joined the basketball team and hung out with a new group of friends. I saw less of him as we progressed through school, and it was disheartening.

My nightmares returned and bled over into reality. I felt like I was underwater and couldn't surface. I quit reaching out for anyone or anything. I couldn't breathe, and I turned inside and closed my eyes. There were days when Mom called me from sleep to the table for dinner, and I'd have no recollection of having gone to school or even a string of memories from the previous week. I noticed that voices seemed muffled, but I didn't care to hear what they were saying. It appeared as if a fog drifted between every other person and me, so I stopped trying to see their faces.

By March, I'd lost weight and was thinner than usual. To Mom, I had all the symptoms of mononucleosis. She questioned the morality of my activities at school, and it insulted me. Her inquisition about my involvement with girls outside the church angered me. She took me to the doctor's office for an examination and a blood draw, and the results came back negative. Dad tried to dig inside my heart but followed the same path as Mom with assumptions and accusations. I didn't know what was wrong with me. By the time they finished, I wanted to tell them I had engaged in sin. I wanted a girl to be close to, hell, any female would suffice, but there was no one bound to me, not a single soul. If there were such things as being tied to apron strings and coattails, this ridiculous incident severed the connection; I closed the door to my parents.

Carrie invited me to her house on weekends and I looked forward to the time, but she couldn't afford it. Two babies occupied her, and I didn't want to be a third. I spent hours walking the lanes between the fields. I went down to the creek where I used to catch fish in the traps that Dad helped me make. I sat on the rocks and watched the swallows drop from their mud nests under the bridge. Their aerial display mesmerized me. I remembered being on the farm before Joe had his initial seizure and recalled Danny's first rabbit hunt in the west field with a shotgun Dad bought him for Christmas. I thought about the weekend cookouts where Carrie grilled more chicken than anyone could eat and the Sundays after dinner, sitting by the same stream, not yet preoccupied by attending a church that did its best to instill a fear of damnation in me. I realized the swallows, skimming the creek's surface, were most likely the offspring of the birds I observed when I first came here. The feeling that they'd fared so much more beautifully than we had made me cry.

#

In May, the rains came. They fell gently with no angle and felt like a lover whispering in your ear and kissing your cheek. On a gray morning, I woke to get ready for school and found a note on the counter. It was in Dad's handwriting, and it instructed me to stay home and that Brother Charlie would pick me up.

Brother Charlie, one of Dad's church buddies, was a grizzled old veteran of World War II. He was squat and sinewy, with tattoos on his forearms, and a hand missing most of its fingers. Dad liked him; they usually worked shoulder to shoulder at the church site and compared notes on all the tackle they couldn't afford at the Boat, Sport, and Travel Show.

I got dressed and sat in the living room, not knowing what to expect. A few minutes later, Charlie pulled his old Ford truck, with a bass boat in tow, into the drive and honked its horn. I zipped up my sweatshirt and trotted out into the rain. Charlie saw me as he rounded the nose of his rig and hollered, "Are you ready to go fishin'?"

Confused, I asked, "Why are we goin' fishing?"

Charlie pulled his hat off, blinked up into the rain, rubbed his mangled hand on his chin, looked back at me, and said, "Cause it's raining the kind of way that makes fish bite."

He asked, "You got a rain jacket?"

I told him I didn't, and he said, "Well, I been wet quite a few times too."

I still wasn't sure why this was happening, but it was as exciting as sneaking out of a window at night.

We drove to Morse Reservoir, where Charlie showed me how to put a boat in the water and pick up someone from the shore. Once we were both in the ship, he twisted the Evinrude's throttle and we motored across the lake to what he called his "honey hole." As we approached the site, Charlie brought the engine down to an idle and asked me to move to the bow and watch for snags. He cut the motor, and we drifted up under some overhanging branches.

He dropped the anchor, arranged a tin bucket full of live minnows, passed me a rod with a spinning reel, and said, "We're just gonna sit here for a minute and let the fish get to know us."

The rain on the water sounded like heavy breathing. I was thinking about being wet when Charlie pressed a metal thermos lid of hot coffee against my arm. I took it and thanked him. After swallowing a few mouthfuls, I passed it back to him, and he finished it. Charlie picked up his line, grabbed a minnow from the bucket, and ran his hook through its wriggling tail. I followed suit, and we cast our bait between the boat and the bank.

Charlie let out a low whistle and whispered, "This oughta be a goodun."

It wasn't more than a few seconds before the fish pulled our bobbers under the surface. Every time we reeled in our lines, we had crappies that were larger than Charlie's intact hand. More often than not, they hit our bait before the floats touched their stops. With each fish, Charlie howled, "Boy, I tell ya what!"

In little more than two hours, we stacked two stringers with fish. With a wide grin, Charlie exclaimed, "Boy, I tell ya what, we're slayin' 'em today!"

I proudly confirmed his assessment, and he noted the clothes I was wearing didn't have a dry stitch to them.

He blew out another low whistle and admitted, "Well, I reckon we'd better leave a few for some other fellers." We packed the poles under the gunnels, pulled the stringers into the boat, and headed back to the launch.

After loading the boat and strapping down the tackle, we headed east toward Anderson. The rain was still falling along Strawtown Road as Charlie navigated the sweeping turns that cut their way through fields waking from the winter.

Over the sound of the windshield wipers, Charlie asked, "How's yer brothers doin'?"

I felt a pinch in my gut and responded, "I reckon they're doing as good as they can."

I turned my head to the window and searched the horizon, grudgingly expecting further questions about their condition.

After a pause, Charlie asked, "How are you doin'?"

I wasn't expecting a question so pointed. In the seven years since we moved to Anderson, no one had ever asked me about my wellbeing. His query made me choke. I knew I wasn't doing well, but I couldn't string those words together. Being confronted confused me. If I'd turned to meet his eyes, I'd have cried, so I kept my face to the window.

I mustered two words, "I'm doin'."

I felt he had my heart in his hand, and after a lengthy pause, he said, "Most of the time, the hardest part of anything is the doin'."

After an equally long pause, I faced him, and we nodded at each other.

Charlie asked no further questions on the way to the house. There was a comfortable silence that rested between us. With twelve simple words and a nod, I realized that Charlie cared about me and somehow understood what was going on inside me.

When we pulled into the drive, I thanked him for taking me fishing and opened the truck's door.

He said, "Don't run off; we gotta get your fish!"

He met me at the back of the truck, pulled out a stringer, handed it over, and said, "The river ought to be good for fishing in a few weeks, if you'd like to go—you ever fished a river?"

I hadn't, and the idea sounded like fun.

I said, "Brother Charlie, I'd like that a lot."

He put his mangled hand on my shoulder and said, "You ain't gotta call me that—you call me Charlie, and I'll call you when the river is ready."

I smiled and thanked him. Charlie backed his fishing rig out of the driveway and headed down the road. I noticed Mom's car in the garage when I walked around the house to gather a bucket of water for the fish. I stowed the stringer near the service door and went inside to get a knife. Mom stopped me in the kitchen and asked if my trip was successful. I was still standoffish from weeks before and grudgingly admitted I'd caught some. She suggested I change into dry clothes. I told her it was raining, and I needed to clean the catch before they got slimy. She rushed toward the sink, grabbed a mixing bowl, and made a saltwater bath to soak them. I mentioned I could pack them in the freezer, but she said she wanted to fry them for dinner.

I went outside, pulled fish out of the bucket, and processed them. I felt terrible for not wanting to talk to Mom, and I was angry for feeling that way. I recognized it wasn't Charlie's idea to take me fishing; it was most likely Dad's plan, and Mom was also in on it. I figured they had used Charlie to bridge the gap between us.

I initiated the forming of our chasm, and it disgusted me. I understood a ridiculous burden weighed on Mom and Dad. I didn't call for any attention from them; I never asked for anything because I refused to add to their struggle. I tried to be as small as possible and not make a ripple or even a shadow. I didn't intend to be under their light, but somehow—unconsciously—I betrayed myself and exhibited a signal. I failed to fathom what was wrong with me other than possibly having a brain tumor. Like a pack mule off its lead, I couldn't grasp what harnessed me, but I wanted out from under it, and the only thing that seemed to ease the strain was running. By now, the only work I was halfway decent at was being distant, and I thought it best to hold my course.

I flipped handfuls of gore into the garden bed and slipped the fish carcasses into the bowl of saltwater. I finished my task by the light from the kitchen window and shivered from the rain.

#

As summer pulled out things that slept in the ground, I went fishing on the river with Charlie. We waded along the bank off Moss Island Road behind the old meatpacking plant. Charlie said the fish in there were fat from sucking up blood and offal from the factory discharge drains. He taught me how to seine for bait with a net strung between two sticks. We saved the crayfish I caught, ripped their claws off, ran hooks through their tails, and cast them to the center of the turbulence. Charlie was wrong about the size of the fish we reeled to the shallows. They weren't fat; they were monsters. Usually, they broke our lines.

We went fishing at least one day a week. I liked to watch Charlie in moving water. On land, he waddled with a bow-legged gait from arthritic knees, but when wading through the river, he moved as if he were a boy. The tattoos coloring his arms were blurry from age. He told me he got them during World War II, somewhere in the Pacific. Sometimes he walked out, up to his waist in the heavy current, staring downstream and whispering to something unseen while rubbing those indigo marks with his mangled hand. The first few instances worried me, and I'd call to him, asking if he was okay. It shook him from his spell, and he'd say he was fine and that he just remembered something. When I interrupted him, he'd back out of the depths and resume his angling. He could have been praying—it wasn't uncommon for the church people to pray anywhere—but he looked engaged with things just out of sight. I asked him about the war on the drives back to the house, but he'd say he couldn't recall much as it was so long ago.

After several excursions, I gained enough courage to ask him about the fingers missing from his hand, and in his fashion of using as few words as possible, he said, "Haw, I did something stupid—didn't need 'em anyway."

#

Charlie had several character-filled fishing buddies, but my favorite was Sister Hazel. She hailed from ancestral property deep in the mountains of eastern Tennessee. Hazel was a featherweight, but what she lacked in dimensions crossed the air between you and made you warm. She was old-timey and steeped in backwoods religion, but she didn't ply you with it or try to make you feel bad. Her high-collared dresses skimmed the ground, but they never stopped her from wading in the river with Charlie and me. Even though advanced in age, she was firm and had a quality that gave me the impression she had many more years than I yet to live. I had a hard time meeting her gaze. Hazel's dazzling eyes did more than shine; they searched my soul. When she talked with me, she palmed my cheek and rested the pad of her thumb under my eye. Like a Whisperer, she peered inside me. Once she had my eyes, I can't say if she said anything; her lips moved, but there was another language I heard, and it was peaceful. She often claimed to hold my arm for support, but it seemed more so out of affection.

During each vernal and autumnal equinox, Sister Hazel visited her hollow in the Appalachian Mountains. I'm sure she had several things to maintain at her property, but it appeared as if her crucial task was as a bootlegger of water. Toward the solstices, she rolled back to Indiana in her vintage Oldsmobile that rocked and swayed under a heavy load. She packed every nook and cranny of that car with a diverse assortment of plastic and glass vessels filled with the effluence from a spring that flowed through her land. She swore by its medicinal traits and wouldn't drink any other liquid. She bestowed gallon jugs or quart jars on a few fortunate people. She was right; I'd never tasted water of more excellent quality.

#

In between fishing trips with Charlie, I attended drivers' education classes, baled hay for Davis Dairy in the fields west of Anderson, and maintained my daily chores. Even though I felt reasonably invisible at home, I didn't like being there. Joe crept around the house like an angry bear and growled at most anything. He'd never been agreeable, but that had always been a quality he—and everyone else—thought comical. Now, the combination of surgeries, painkillers, and steroids turned him sour and mouthy. He seemed to hover near the edge of rage and needed coaxing away from violent outbursts. His eyes were glassy and disconnected. Living exhausted him.

#

I kicked around with Burly, a buddy from junior high. The frame of his body shaped him like a sheet of plywood. He was a fantastic athlete and seemed to be mostly lungs. He dominated distance running and regularly ran fifteen miles from Lapel to Chesterfield—where he'd dominate in a 5K race—and then run back to Lapel. His love of illuminating human quirks was as fanatical as his training regimen, and his laugh was infectious.

We knew each other in elementary school, but we didn't connect until junior high when our schedules shunted us into art and music classes. Technically, art and music were electives—if you had an interest in exploring your creative side—but more often than not, the administration forcibly filled most of the seats with underachievers and misfits such as Burly and myself. Everyone in attendance was an easy target for Burly. He assessed us as a school of fish trying to swim upstream without getting wet, and it drove him silly. He couldn't help himself from wryly poking or grandstanding anyone's slightest mistake or embarrassment. I don't believe he intended any harm; I think he didn't want to feel alone. We were fortunate to have him, because he brought comedy to our grindingly dull incarceration.

We played JV football for two seasons but didn't progress beyond the special teams. After incurring injuries from a poorly planned practice, we spent several games on the bench. When the coach tasked us with being water boys, I dropped off the team.

Burly and I traded weekends staying at each other's house. On Sundays, he went along with me to church. It was nice to have an uncompromised confidant in attendance to help me shoulder the religious culture's weight. Just as he did at school, he brought levity to the situation. He thought the church's spectacle was entertaining but noted the opulence of the sanctuary; he questioned the lavish spending on the structure by stating its current use for Christian activities needed scrapping to accommodate a live performance by Van Halen. The parishioners targeted him for salvation, but everyone—by Burly's standards—was a little too friendly for his taste, so he eventually stopped spending his weekends with me.

#

Winter settled in, and Lamech came home on leave for Christmas. He brought me a set of Army fatigues (Battle Dress Uniform or BDU) and a pair of jungle boots. It was the first time he'd ever willingly given me anything, and this simple act honored me. For the first time since we were little, I felt as if he liked me. He asked if I could take him camping, and I gladly agreed.

There wasn't any snow on the ground, but it was frozen. After I gathered my old survival kit and borrowed a tent from Whitey, we headed across the field to my woods. We set up a camp close to the big beech tree and built a small fire. We shared the remaining C rations from Uncle Bill and a partial package of hotdogs. The firelight's glow captured our breath, the occasional falling leaf, and nearby branches. Lamech told me stories of Army life and weapons he used in training. He described Oktoberfest, carnivals in Germany, and trips by train to Spain and France. He spoke more that night than ever before. He continued sharing until the fire dwindled and the dying wind let frost settle on the surrounding earth. We climbed into our shelter and slept fitfully.

I woke well before dawn with a powerful urge to piss. There was ice in the tent's interior from our respiration, and I couldn't feel my feet as they were numb from the cold. Lamech awakened with my stirrings. He said he was sick and claimed it was from rotten hot dogs. He asked if I could build another fire for us. I went out and stumbled through the underbrush to urinate and collect fallen branches. By the time I got a flame going, I had recognized my toes by the pain under my nails. I slapped my hands together and blew on them to get the feeling back. Lamech eventually crawled out of the tent and wandered off in the dark to puke. When he returned, we decided to break camp and head home. I pulled the shelter down and rolled everything into it while Lamech warmed himself. We scattered the fire, kicked dirt over the embers, and quietly walked out of the woods into the field.

The view was breathtaking. A brilliant moon illuminated a heavy frost covering the corn stubble and gave it a magical appearance. I wondered at the spectacle as Lamech shivered with cold and clutched his gut on the long walk home. We crept in through the garage, and Lamech went to Tonya's room while I crawled into my bed and surrendered to sleep.

After the holidays, Lamech, Tonya, and their daughter packed their belongings and left for Germany. The absence of Lamech's family made the house seem empty. Again, I felt as if I was adrift and sinking. The world around me went dark.

#

By March, Mom and Dad had taken me for another CT scan, but the results were negative. Still, it was grim, like someone forcefully twisting your mandible into your maxilla, and all you can do is listen to your teeth grind and fracture. At each instance, we expected to find a brain tumor—maybe next time we would. These appointments took everything out of me.

I'd given up feeling any resentment toward Mom and Dad. I'd given up feeling most anything. When the rains came, I found another note on the counter with orders to skip school and go fishing with Charlie. When Charlie arrived at the house with his rig, he wasn't alone; Dad rolled into the driveway and parked next to him. It confounded me; I'd never witnessed Dad leave work early unless Joe or Danny was in trouble. I met them at the door as they were coming inside. I asked Dad if something was wrong and he answered that everything was just fine. He pitched a packaged poncho at me and jokingly offered that he'd skipped school. Charlie took off his hat and sat in the kitchen as Dad made coffee to fill his thermos. We waited while he changed clothes and gathered up his old Zebco reel and logging jacket. The three of us slid onto Charlie's truck's vinyl bench seat and headed out to Morse Reservoir.

Dad and Charlie enjoyed being together and every time they met, they chatted up and down as if they hadn't seen each other in years. Charlie contained a volume of simple truths and wisdom that Dad was keen to discuss. With one another, the age seemed to peel off them. Their personalities brightened as if they shared an elixir of healing. Being with them affected me as well; I didn't know there was a comfort I missed. Sitting shoulder to shoulder between Charlie and Dad stirred feelings within me; it was like an old friend coming through your door or hearing a familiar voice in a storm. Memories of sitting with Unck and his brothers around Mamaw's kitchen table came and threatened to wet my eyes. It was like taking a breath after being underwater for too long or narrowly escaping a calamity.

Charlie, Dad, and I skipped a day of school at least every other week. One of their mutual friends, Brother Raymond, started joining us on our fishing trips. Raymond wouldn't let me call him anything but Ray. Ray was a veteran of World War II. He was quiet, if not stoic, and only spoke to illuminate Dad's or Charlie's foibles or to acknowledge—in single-word sentences—when a condition was beautiful, peaceful, or perfect. Ray made me feel like I was standing next to an invulnerable tree that had been tested by the turbulence of innumerable storms; the winds, unable to wrench its branches and roots, had finally left it alone. One of his shoulders was a little lower than the other, and its hand wasn't used for much other than small things like baiting a hook, tying a line, or balancing a cup of coffee while he worked at something. If I was in Ray's vicinity—in Charlie's boat, on the bank of the river or pond, or walking into a bait shop—his good arm was around my shoulder and the world in front of us was, as Ray would say, "Perfect."

#

Summer settled in, and Dad hired me to help maintain the grounds at Universal Tool. I didn't mind the long hours of mowing and painting as I earned more money than I ever did cutting lawns around the neighborhood. Danny's seizures still hit him in clusters, and he couldn't drive, so the three of us rode to work together. After my initial week at the tool shop, I gained a new respect for Danny. He'd been experiencing at least one seizure a day, and they slammed into him as if he'd stumbled into the path of a fast-moving truck. It didn't matter how many convulsions he had—they were each as frightening and heartbreaking as the first. To prevent serious injury, Dad refused to let Danny operate any machinery, and it wounded both of them. Danny worked with the engineers on assembling research projects—which he enjoyed—but he ground his teeth when he had to hand over a part to another machinist for modifications. He was as volatile as ever but now seemed focused on his condition and not the world. I admired him for his determination. He wasn't a quitter, not by any means.

After Dad checked the locks on all the buildings at the end of each day, we headed north to Anderson. Danny, wrung out from his struggle, was usually asleep before we merged into traffic on the interstate. Dad was glad to be heading home and was talkative, but several things strained our relationship, and it wasn't his shortcoming. He tried to close the distance between us, but it must have been like crawling through brambles. I wanted him but didn't feel I needed him. Maybe it was good I was resistant to responding; after a few days of trying to get me to talk, he reminisced or vented.

He spoke of his childhood and the struggles that resided there. He shared how he felt about his abusive father and his loving mother. He talked about their shack and shivering under sheets as the wind blew snow through the house. He laughed at memories of splitting kindling and purposefully cutting off the tip of his brother's thumb with a hatchet. He chuckled about his little sister stealing squirrels from the cat for dinner. He described gnawing on fried chicken feet as if they were a delicacy instead of a stopgap to stave off hunger. He recalled being shut out of his home after his mother died and crying himself to sleep outside in the night. He waxed emotional over the old souls from town that looked over him by providing odd jobs and occasional meals. He mulled over Garnna's death, Padanaram, and force-feeding Shelam to keep her alive. He poured out his worry for Danny and Joe and wondered if he was the cause of all the grief that had befallen us. Like a modern-day Job, he questioned if this was a wager played between Lucifer and God. If I could have spoken, there was nothing I could say.

#

By the end of August, I had my driver's license, and I'd earned enough money to buy Carrie's old Chevette. On Fridays, I drove to the farm to help her and Ted bale straw or mow the lanes. Except for church, I was free to do as I pleased on the weekends. I spent most of my time driving on county roads and listening to mixtapes I made from Ted's 1960s and 1970s LP collection. Buffalo Springfield, Jefferson Airplane, The Moody Blues, and The Eagles dominated my stereo.

The summer before, I adopted an acoustic guitar that Dad had squirreled away in his closet. I played it every day—learning by ear—and was fairly proficient. I wanted an electric guitar and scoured the *Trader Classified Paper* for a suitable candidate. I found a 1976 Gibson Les Paul for four hundred dollars. I had two hundred dollars in my pocket and was afraid the deal would get away from me. I asked Dad if he'd be willing to go half on it with me, and he agreed. After bringing the electrified gem home, I set myself toward practicing Led Zeppelin's foundational riffs. Hendrix's licks were a greater challenge, and they kept me occupied while shut in my room at night. I still had to hide my music from my parents and the church; I played through a small effects box and headphones that came with the purchase and hid my tapes in my jacket pockets.

#

Shortly before my junior year, Burly came rolling around in a battered truck with mismatched wheels and a manual shifter on the column. The steering wheel made a complete revolution before the machine decided to change direction, the brakes worked most of the time, and the fuel gauge was nonexistent.

The beater was a vehicular Frankenstein and was nowhere near roadworthy, but the terror of driving it was high comedy.

Burly was dating his long-time pursuit, RaAnn Parks. Since junior high, we'd all been around each other and shared the same knack of art and humor. Ra was the only girl in school who looked me in the eye and asked pointed questions about my behavior. I figured she enjoyed making fun of me. She kept her hair cut and curled in a short bob and lined her eyes and lips like the girls in a John Hughes film. She was thin, fast, and bright. Like holding a vial of nitroglycerin, it was exciting to be next to her.

That autumn, the three of us participated in decorating the juniors' hallway for the homecoming competitions. We spent weeknights at the school, crafting our theme on enormous sheets of paper laid out on the hall floor. As the nights progressed, Ra's work edged closer to mine. Her questions about my clothes, queries about the things I liked, and praise for my craftsmanship were noticeably forward. It reminded me of an Art Club trip to Nashville, Indiana, where she slid next to me on the bus's bench seat, clutched my arm, and rested her hand on the inside of my thigh. Then, I figured she was playing with me, but now she seemed sincere, and it was flattering.

On the fourth evening of homecoming events, I drove to meet the two of them at Burly's. His mom said he was with Ra, so I headed to her house. Ra answered the door when I knocked and said she hadn't seen Burly since the afternoon. I asked if she wanted a ride to the school, and she suggested a trip to McDonald's on the way. During the drive to Edgewood, we laughed about everyday things. Heading back to Lapel, she leaned against me and found sport in pressing french fries into my mouth. *My god, she was cute!* I couldn't believe she was so close to me. Her face was inches from mine. She didn't flinch when I drifted into the gravel on the side road.

After rolling into the school parking lot, Ra suggested we skip work since Burly's truck wasn't there. To Ra's frustration, I cruised by the few places I expected to find him. As the sun set, I pulled into the gravel along her home to let her out. She had both of her hands wrapped around my arm and gave me the impression she didn't want to let go. I didn't want her to let go, but she wasn't mine. We walked down to Burly's and knocked on his door, but no one answered. By now it was dark. We made our way back to her house, making jokes about our oddly shaped shadows cast by the streetlamps. We played in the light until it was past my curfew. Eventually I headed to Anderson, knowing she wanted me but also understanding she was committed to a relationship with Burly.

By the time homecoming was over, I'd pissed off Burly. Justifiably so. We'd stopped talking to one another, and our passing in the hallways was tense. I couldn't get Ra out of my mind. To complicate matters, whenever she called, I'd meet her. On weekends, she worked at an antique store in Anderson, where I'd take her milkshakes and french fries. She'd sit on the counter and wrap her legs around my waist while she munched on her treats. We talked about subjects we liked and didn't like. She inquired about the church I attended and my family. She asked questions about situations I'd tried to forget or ignore, but not in a way to satisfy her curiosity; it seemed she wanted to be part of my story. I felt fully ensnared by her, and I didn't want her to let me go.

#

One night, late in the autumn, I woke, believing that someone had called my name. I held my breath and intently listened, but the only voice I could hear was a cricket at my window.

I tried to go back to sleep, but my mind was stirring. I felt as if there was something I should know or remember, but I couldn't tie a thought to it, and it was vexing. I lay there listening and searching until I heard Dad making coffee in the kitchen. Mom joined him, and they quietly conversed until they both left for work. I failed to make heads or tails of what I was feeling, so I got dressed and sat outside until I had to leave for school. The experience dug at me throughout the day.

That evening, I learned that my fishing buddy, Sister Hazel, had died. It was hurtful, knowing I'd never again feel her hand on my arm or look into her eyes. Paying out line, trying to catch something to assuage my feelings, I remembered the event the night before and wondered if that was Hazel speaking my name. If there was magic in the world, she would be one to hold it. I found comfort in the thought that maybe in her passing, she'd said goodbye.

#

It was Friday night, and I had a mandatory youth function to attend in Sheridan. There was a bonfire and several denim-clad girls standing nearby. At first it seemed it might not be a bad experience, but it quickly turned into an abysmal affair. The pastor began to rail against science. He claimed Satan planted dinosaur bones in the earth to mislead Man from the teachings of God. Since there was no record of God creating such creatures, the only available solution must be some sort of deception by demonic forces. Ted and Carrie were in attendance, but she was in a nasty mood and angry with him. I felt very much alone. I quit the fire midservice, got in my car, and drove away.

The night air was frigid. There would be frost in the morning. I rolled down my window to feel the wind on my face. I hoped it would remedy the feelings left by the departure of

Sister Hazel and clear my head of the stupidity I'd just experienced. It was troublesome seeing Carrie angry. I was feeling
down, which seemed to be how I was most of the time. I'd
attempted to avoid Ra and Burly for the past few weeks, and it
darkened me. I didn't want to go home, but I had no place to
go. I turned south off State Road 38 and meandered through
Hamilton County until I found myself in Lapel. I made a few
passes up and down Main Street, drove out through the cemetery, and cruised around the school.

　　I didn't want to be alone. I was so lonely; it seemed to ache
under my skin. I drove by Burly's and parked alongside Ra's
home. I walked up to the front door and knocked on the glass.
I was cold—cold on the inside—and I wanted to feel warm.
After several seconds, I turned my back to the house and was
about to step off the porch when the door swung open. I spun
around to find Ra, as cute as ever, reaching to pull me indoors.
We made our way through the darkened halls to the kitchen.
We sat facing each other in chairs at the counter. She unzipped
my jacket and slipped her hands around my waist. She said
she liked the way I smelled—like a campfire. I told her where
I'd been, and its depressing nature. I shared with her the passing of sister Hazel and the premonition I'd had the previous
night. She asked a ledger of questions about me. She laid her
head against my chest, and I wrapped my arms around her. We
remained that way for a long time. Her hair smelled sweet, and
it was soft and smooth against the corner of my mouth.

　　Her parents—opening the front door—roused us, and we
quietly slipped out the back of the house. We walked to my
car, where I opened the door and backed into the driver's seat.
She crouched just outside the opening. Instinctively, we leaned
close to one another. I looked into her moss-colored eyes and
inhaled her breath. We pressed our foreheads together and followed with our lips.

#

The following week at school was troublesome. The cold war between Burly and me was about to boil over. I expected a fistfight at every instance of passing him in the halls. I also anticipated warmth from Ra, but she seemed distant.

#

Another week passed. Most of my calls to Ra went unanswered and when I spoke with her, she was guarded and quiet. The following Saturday, I thought of visiting her at the antique store. I mulled it over most of the morning, trying to formulate an excuse to drive there, uninvited. After noon, she surprised me by entering the house without knocking and slipping into my bedroom. She was neatly attired in a fitted white blouse and a short plaid skirt. She perfectly exposed her well-formed knees from below the hem of her skirt to the top of her white knee socks. She removed her gold hoop earrings and laid them on my drawing table. Her saddle oxfords left no prints on the carpet as she crossed the room and kneeled in front of me as I sat on my bed. I told her I'd missed her and asked why she'd come.

Quietly dismissive, she said, "I wanted to see you." Her focus was singularly on my eyes, and her hands were on my knees. We leaned our heads together and kissed. After a moment, she leaned away. I noticed her eyes on other facets of me. She looked me over as if I were something she wanted to remember.

With purpose, she stood up and looked around my room, turned back, and said, "I have to go."

Somehow I knew she meant more than leaving my house, but I didn't want to believe it. I walked her out and helped her into her car. She closed the door with no further words, backed out of the driveway, and drove away. I returned to my room, where I noticed her earrings on my table. They held traces of her perfume. I put them in my jacket pocket, excited by having a reason to meet her again.

On Monday, at school, Ra had her arms around another boy, and it wasn't Burly. It was hurtful to see, but there wasn't anything I could do. I rolled her earrings in my palm and knew there was no point in returning them. Like a little house wren, she'd flitted toward me, turned, and flew away.

Burly saw it too. I don't know if she spoke to him in parting, but his defenses eventually gave way. Like a storm blowing out, it was quiet between us. I'd wounded him, and although we'd never be as close as before, we had fresh ground with each other; being hurt by the same girl bonded us in a loss. We both took it in problematic ways. Burly dropped out of sports and seemed to drift on the fringes of the social circles while I embraced the loneliness I'd been feeling, enveloped myself in music, and went through my daily motions—spiritless.

#

The power and frequency of the seizures debilitated Danny. His tumor had grown to an alarming size and was moving into both hemispheres of his brain. The only option was surgery, and the procedure was more than grim; it might permanently disable, if not kill him.

On the third morning of November 1987, our extended family sat in a cramped waiting room as Danny—in the surgery ward—received a spinal block and a local anesthetic at multiple points along his hairline. For the next six hours, he remained conscious as the surgeon pressed a scalpel through the skin above his brow and peeled back a palm-sized flap of the scalp. Danny felt the pressure and listened to a craniotome's whine as it ground its way through his skull to remove a section from his frontal lobe. He responded to requests to speak, answer questions, and move various parts of his body as the specialist inserted spatulas, forceps, and microknives at areas circumnavigating the nest of cancer at the center of his brain. Throughout the procedure, Danny suffered convulsions and wept at the horror.

Near the end of the surgery, we were all spent but didn't appear nearly as wrought as the surgeon when he walked into the waiting room and called us to the consultation office.

The surgeon considered the action a success; he believed he had removed the entire tumor with Danny incurring minimal damage. It did affect his vocal and motor skills on his left side, so he'd need speech and physical therapy to recover. It sounded challenging but promising to think Danny might be able to function like a healthy human being.

In pairs, we went to visit Danny in the recovery room. He was still sedated and his complexion was milky, like the white gauze and tape that encapsulated his head. His eyelids were greasily translucent, and I could see the shape of his irises behind them. His mouth was agape, and stubble surrounded his chin as if he'd been out of circulation for several days. I didn't want to see him like this. I didn't need to be part of the parade to view the spectacle, but what else was there to do? Everything about our situation disgusted me, but I stood there, with everyone—our hands held to a fire—crying for a remedy or release.

#

I'd ruined the clutch of the Chevette while abusing the roads between Lapel and home—it was for sale in the front yard, as the cost to repair it was more than it was worth. I'd asked permission to drive Mom's Dodge Charger to visit Burly. He and I didn't have a plan for this Saturday night other than being out on the road.

The stock Chrysler stereo couldn't amplify my pirated copy of *Physical Graffiti* enough to drown out the growl in my mind. I didn't want to think about Danny's surgery and how it left him or feel my shame for not wanting to do so. I pressed the pedal to the floor and shot past Weeks's Marathon into the rain. The headlights isolated a forty-foot stretch of inky black road and captured leaves tumbling across its surface in the November wind. When I entered Lapel, I cut the wheel and skidded onto Main Street, sloppily navigated a few turns, and came to a sliding stop in the gravel drive along Burly's house.

Burly ran out from the cover of the porch and jumped into the passenger seat. He was high and giggling. From his jacket, he pulled a bag of weed with a few twisted joints. He'd copped the dope from a coworker at Captain D's seafood shop where he worked. He split open the Ziploc pouch, stuffed a joint between his lips, and lit it. He offered it to me, and I readily inhaled as deeply as I could, hoping it would stand up to its promise. I didn't immediately feel anything, but I feigned euphoria, cackled out a forced laugh, stabbed the gas pedal, and launched out of Lapel back toward Anderson. Burly tried to turn up the stereo, but its digital readout wouldn't go any higher than 26. Robert Plant wailed through the speakers, "... Everybody needs the light!" as we passed the roach back and forth.

I slowed the car as we rolled into Anderson's blighted heart, over the tracks near the Wigwam, and down the slope toward Mounds Mall. I finally felt the weed's full effect, but all I could hear was Unck in my head telling me, "Don't you mess around with that stuff or I'll jerk a knot in your tail!"

We strolled through the mall, wielding our insobriety as if it was a badge of courage. We followed gaggles of girls, thinking our bumbling swagger might entice them to be interested in us, but we were too high to register any engagement if there was any. We satiated our boredom inside Woolworth's, looking at goldfish and hamsters.

Burly bought a Pink Floyd cassette—*The Wall*—and after a few more laps inside the mall, we retreated to the car. Burly fumbled with the cellophane around his newly purchased album and grew nervous as it didn't list the songs he expected.

He cried, "Fuck! Is this half an album?"

He giggled and mocked a possible disclaimer, "Pink Floyd's real sorry they couldn't fit all the songs on this tape—you'll have to spend another twenty dollars for the rest of them."

With anger, he jammed the cassette into the stereo, and for the first time, I heard, "... So you thought you might like to go to the show..." and it enraptured me to hear a sound similar to the one playing in the background of my thoughts. Burly lit up another joint, and we crept back toward Lapel along 32 as the rain fell heavily and drowned out the rest of the night.

Broken Teeth/Angry Young Man

I was sick the winter of my junior year. I had several fevers and sinus infections, and my jaw constantly burned from my wisdom teeth slowly fracturing my molars. Mom bought me a leather jacket for Christmas, and I promptly painted a picture of an angry hound with a gun on the back of it and three letters at its base—DOG. I smoked a lot of weed with Burly and consumed bottles of overpriced booze from the school's black market.

The hurt and hate I'd been feeling was like a slime of mud on a footpath; I got more of it on me the further I walked. It felt better to stab blame at everything I didn't want to deal with and the facts I couldn't change. Like digging at a scab or pressing on a toothache, the hate felt better than hurt. Hate felt good. It was easy to hate Ra for dumping me. It was easy to hate Mom and Dad for not being around, and it was easy to hate the church for hell. It was easy to hate Joe and Danny for exhibiting what I would be. It was easy to hate myself for being me.

I was unmoored again, registering no sense of direction or time. If the sun was in the sky, it didn't seem to shine, and night settled just after noon. I bought a set of headphones and spent many hours listening to music and walking in the fields around the house.

#

Without a car, I rode the bus to and from school. Every day, I sat by myself in the back with my head to the window and monitored the passing terrain.

At some point, Shelly, an ornery minx, dropped onto my bench and asked, "What—outside that window—is so vexing?"

I responded, "Why are you in my seat?"

She placed her palm on the inside of my leg, slid it up to cup my crotch, and said, "I'm just so horny, and you're so hot, I can't resist myself!" With that, she buckled over with laughter but kept her hand on my thigh.

Shelly was short, slim, and smart. She was always a few steps ahead of everyone and didn't have a problem making sure they understood that fact. She'd square off against anyone and cut them down with a brace of surgically applied words. Their only defense was to slink away, wounded because Shelly—somehow—knew their darkest fears. Although she was quick and potentially ruthless, there seemed to be a vulnerable tenderness under her shell. She had an older brother, and they lived in a wooded subdivision with their grandmother. Shelly never mentioned her parents, so I figured it was best I didn't ask about them. She was keen to sit next to me. Each morning and in the afternoons, Shelly saved a place for me. She enjoyed resting her hand on the inside of my thigh as much as I did hers, but that's as sensual as we ever were; it was a comedy, but there was a small comfort.

One afternoon, Shelly alerted me she would be driving her grandmother's car to school the next day. I asked if she could pick me up on the way but she cut me off, saying she had other plans. As expected, Shelly wasn't on the bus the following morning. Oddly, she was absent during the first period. Sometime around my second class, the receptionist summoned me to the office and informed me that my sister was picking me up for an appointment. It confused me; Carrie picking me up—for something I didn't know about—made no sense. About the time I sat down at the school's front door, a yellow Cadillac rolled up to the sidewalk. Its passenger window descended to expose Shelly's tiny body at the steering wheel. I blinked a few times before I realized she was waving for me to get in the coach. After looking over my shoulder, I exited the foyer and walked out to the Cadillac. She leaned over, cackling, and breathlessly proclaimed that the office ladies were a bunch of rubes and that today, she was my sister. She called me a dummy, too, and motioned for me to get inside. We spent the day at Castleton Mall, and once a week, until she graduated, we skipped school in the same fashion.

#

Tree peepers, calling in the night from the swamps, heralded the return of spring. It seemed as if I hadn't heard them since grade school. Their chorus was sweet and soothing. I remembered this was the time of year for catching tadpoles, rooting my feet in the earth with mud between my toes, and standing under a new sun.

The following Saturday, I followed a muddy track to a rise between the field stubble. In the distance, where the cattails rose some yards short of the water, I saw a figure with a five-gallon bucket, stooped and running their hands through the muck. I was wary at the prospect of a stranger milling around in an area I considered my personal property. I sidestepped into the weeds of the fencerow to hide and crept closer to identify the interloper. Having quietly closed on them, I spied a thick boy through the tall grass—about my age—wearing cutoff denim shorts and a bleached t-shirt.

He was so engaged in collecting bullfrog eggs, he startled when I yelled, "Hey!"

When he irritably responded, "Krieky!" I instantly knew it couldn't be anyone but Toomer. We laughed off the surprise introduction as I slipped off my shoes, squished through the mud to where he was, and joined him in gathering emergent life.

Crayfish had been busy erecting their fortifications, and bird tracks disturbed the smooth surface of the clay. In the bottom of the flooded furrows, clumps of frog eggs and strings of toad eggs clung to debris from past harvests. Schools of tadpoles, already exhibiting transformation, swam from depression to depression. The most prized specimens to collect were the thumb-sized frog pollywogs with green backs and gold bellies. After we filled Toomer's bucket with amphibians, we squeezed through the cordon of cattails and waded in the swamp's deeper portion. We searched for a floating platform that high school boys cobbled together when Toomer and I were in elementary school. The fort was well known, even legendary, but they kept its actual location a secret. Eventually, we found the remains—submerged—turning to earth.

Being worn by the heat, muck, and numerous cuts by cattail stalks, we secured the bucket and took turns carrying it back to his house. We deposited our collection in an enormous aquarium stored in Toomer's garage. When we attempted to move it outside and into his home, it slipped from my hands and smashed on the ground, spilling its contents across the gravel drive. Toomer was crestfallen and I could have cried. We tried to scoop the life from the shards of glass and stone, but most of it was unrecoverable and quickly perished in the sun. Toomer handled the event—as I couldn't have—with measured words and grace.

#

I'd known Toomer since moving to Anderson. His family lived in a white two-story home in the fields on the west side of Lone Oak Road. They were always kind and spoke in full sentences to me as if I were a peer or even part of their family. I had difficulty accepting their attention as I felt inferior, soiled, and as coarse as they weren't. It was shocking to witness a household that was so honestly open and loving. They seemed to know each other's struggles and talked about them openly. They shared finances right along with tastes in music and entertainment. Toomer and his dad collected LPs and 45s and went to concerts together.

Toomer and I had mutual interests in creating and nature, but we hadn't shared much time due to my close relationship with Whitey. He was analytical and stubbornly made sound decisions where I went headlong into everything I shouldn't. He kept his nose clean and refused to curse. I respected him and foolishly feared I might rub off on him. I didn't want him to do the things I did or feel the way I was feeling. I often wondered what it would be like if I were a member of their family, and if I had no memory of mine, I could somehow fit and be as content and joyful as they seemed.

They may not have realized it, but I adopted them and consumed as much time as permitted under their roof. Being with Toomer and his family was solace from my summer work at Universal Tool and a striking contrast to my actual life. I spent ten hours each day in the machine shop's heat and oil fumes, endured hazing from the roughnecks and trash talkers, and returned home with my weary father to have dinner with my worried mother and broken brother. Toomer's place was a guilty pleasure and a well-guarded retreat.

#

Around midsummer, Mom and one of the Sisters from church fixed me up on a blind date with a girl from a Pentecostal congregation in Marion, Indiana. They made the arrangements, and I drove an hour north to meet her parents and take her out to dinner.

Tammy was pretty and, with heels on, she was a little taller than me. The first evening, she wore a pink jumper with a broad lace collar. She suggested going to the mall to walk around. After perusing women's clothing stores until the doors closed, she asked to go to Taco Bell. She bubbled on about her friends at school, her youth group, her daddy's permission to wear makeup when she turned seventeen, and her fondness for fountain drink ice from the machine at Taco Bell. She didn't ask any questions or leave room for me to respond to her statements. As she chomped her way through her third cup of ice, all I could think about was taking her home and driving back to mine. Eventually, I delivered her to her door, shook her hand, and headed out to State Road 9.

My drive home was sublime. The wind, laden with the musk of a summer night, rolled through the windows. I scanned the radio channels and discovered an all-night show somewhere at the end of the AM band. They played long cuts of live Hendrix—that I'd never heard—and endless jams from Iron Butterfly. I turned off the highway and explored the county roads in the general direction of Lone Oak Road.

The next morning, Mom pressed for every detail of my date with Tammy. She was trying not to be giddy with excitement, but she wanted me to have a relationship with this girl. During the interrogation—more than a few times—Mom mentioned her matchmaking partner from Temple Mount and the importance of being a good example for the Sister. I felt she was more interested in impressing the church than in how I thought about a liaison with a stranger.

Unfortunately for Tammy, I continued visiting her for the rest of the summer, not as a love interest but for escape and freedom from home. I behaved callously and lied to her. Not only that, but I also occupied the time she could have spent with her church and friends. I told her I had a 9:00 curfew and religiously returned her to her door by 8:00. I whiled the remaining hours cruising to the park in Lapel to get high with Burly. I might have liked Tammy but since the relationship was my mother's, it was fruitless. Further dampening any opportunity for love to grow, I couldn't stop comparing her to Ra.

#

It excited me to begin my senior year. It was a break from the tool shop and a welcome distraction from my life at home. I couldn't believe I'd made it this far without being held back for my shoddy schoolwork. The uninvolved guidance counselors didn't notice I'd pulled three study hours in my first semester and four in my second. My only scholarly stress was my need to pass the second semester of sophomore algebra; I'd failed it in the two previous years and needed the credit to graduate. I'd scheduled the exact number of credits required to get out of school, and the other classes—U.S. History, English, Speech, and Art IV—were most likely a cinch.

Because of my artistic abilities, the yearbook committee solicited me as a resource. They were a well-connected group of honor society members and socialites. The invite seemed disingenuous; I was at the opposite end of their spectrum. At first, I wasn't interested, but when I found they recruited Toomer and offered to throw in a pass—to free me from attending my study periods—I was ready to be their greatest asset.

#

I reserved my first-hour study period to come down from getting high on the way to school. Old metal windows comprised the entire east wall of the room and permitted an unobstructed view of spectacular autumn sunrises. The only other point of interest that competed with what that facade of glass offered was Ra Parks.

She'd taken a desk near the bank of heaters under the windows. I couldn't help myself from watching her. I still felt hurt, but I wanted her. I wanted her to see me and feel how I felt for her. There was an expectation of rejection—she was dating a big ginger named Colt. She'd dated a few guys since I last talked to her. I missed her. It'd been almost a year since we'd kissed. The thought of being with her or not was like leaping into a chasm.

I stewed over us for more than a few weeks until I made a run at her.

"Fuck it," I said to myself and moved to a vacant desk two rows behind her.

There was a kid seated between us, but I coerced him into trading positions with me. Finally, there I was—less than a few feet from her. I scooted my desk forward until its writing board was inches behind her. She was leaning over her work, with the sun illuminating the fine fuzz that ran up her spine from the gap in her skirt, continued under her half shirt, and blended into her nape's short-cropped hair. She smelled sweet, like washed cotton sheets drying in the sunshine. I said nothing that day or the next—I was breathless being this close to her.

The following Monday, with little to study but fixing the distance between her and me, I doodled in my notebook—faces, feathers, tablature, lyrics, and passages from notable books. After several minutes, a trickle of inspiration found its way through my arm, to my pen, and onto a page. The piece of work was excellent. For a minute or two, I stared at it in wonder, then instinctively wrote, "I miss talking to you." I reached around Ra, laid it over her textbook, leaned back in my seat, and helplessly hoped for a response. She held the notebook for a while before returning it without a word. I opened it to the drawing. Next to the image, she'd written, "Why did you stop?"

Why did I stop? What the hell? That seemed like a cop-out. How could she not know why I stopped? It took a minute before I realized that I didn't ask her a question—I'd made a statement. It didn't matter. She looked at what I'd drawn and responded to my communication. I'd made contact and received a message, like an astronaut's first transmission, after rounding the moon's dark side.

Every other object but Ra seemed to fall away from the room. Trapped near the sunrise by the scheduled hour and the forced silence, we were isolated and alone without anyone to bother us. I didn't know how to verbalize the waterfall of thoughts rushing through my mind, and I didn't want to flush her like a bird from this moment. Like an idiot savant, using a primitive code, I tried to communicate my feelings with brief phrases from songs and books I'd poured over while hiding in the library the previous years. She responded with requests for "more" or stated her mood and what she wanted from the day. We penned elaborate scenarios and fantasies involving endangering ourselves and rescuing one another. We anticipated each response and were quick to edit or turn the stories to our liking. All this happened on the pages of a spiral notebook with a pink cover, an unassuming conduit for our wants and needs. We exchanged the journal multiple times during study hall, but never a word. Sometimes she'd take it with her when the bell rang and we had to go our separate ways. She avoided passing it publicly; she'd send it through her close friend or even a subjugated and angry Colt. When we filled the margins and interior covers, I purchased a college-ruled replacement with a pale blue jacket. I prepared the first page with a sinuous drawing of a predator. We agreed only to use black ink.

#

The autumn seemed vibrant, but it could have been what I was feeling by having a link to Ra. I wanted more of her, but she was still dating Colt. Every Thursday, I drove Mom's car to school, and every Thursday, I asked Ra if I could drive her home from school, but she refused. Watching her climb into Colt's truck at the end of the day was frustrating, but I'd entered this without expectation, so it wasn't hurtful.

Fall break was approaching and I saw it as an opportunity to secure time with Ra. I invited her to my home to watch a movie, and she accepted. On the Tuesday before the break, we left school early and Ra drove us to Lone Oak. On entering the house, I heard Joe snorting with laughter from the den. I asked Ra to wait in my room, and I walked down the hall. I found Joe engaged with an episode of *The Golden Girls*. Now entrenched on the couch, he wasn't about to give up the TV. Not wanting to argue with a bear, I returned to Ra with a new plan. I asked if she'd like to go for a walk in my woods, and she agreed. I pulled my Army fatigues from my closet, handed the pants and a sweatshirt to her, and suggested that she change her skirt as I stepped out of my room and closed the door.

We headed out across the corn stubble of the field under a brilliant sun. She asked about Joe and why he was the way he was. I told her what I knew of him before I was born and all the notable events that reduced him to his current state.

It was easy talking with Ra. With her, everything I'd focused so intently on hiding seemed to pour out of me like a tapped keg. She exhibited none of the woundedness that my story brought out so quickly in others. I didn't have to measure my words or hide my opinions. There was no need to brace her at the end of each revelation or tell her I was okay or undamaged; she took the blast, knowing she'd initiated the charge. After nine years of isolation and imprisonment, I felt that I'd found a peer, if not a partner. Being with her was my ultimate escape.

I directed her to the break in the fence and held the wire for her to pass. After we'd gained our footing under the beech tree's canopy, the golden glow that filtered through its ochre foliage struck us with awe. We walked around the pond and looped back to the edge of the beech, where I sat on the ground and reclined against one of its children to have a full view of the parent tree. Ra wandered under the long branches, picking up seed pods and catching leaves in midair. Eventually she returned, seated herself between my legs, and rested against my chest. The world was quiet, and it was ours but for a chipmunk that made its way along a fallen log to investigate our presence. We remained there, watching the varmint and whispering to each other until the light faded. Before dark, we followed a deer trail to the edge and took a last look into the forest before stepping through the gap and out to the field.

When the house came into view, I noticed my parents' and Carrie's cars in the driveway. The tension inside the house was palpable as Ra and I entered the front door. I could feel something negative, so I asked Ra to wait by the door.

When I walked into the kitchen, Mom, with vitriol, demanded, "Where have you been—whose car is in the driveway—what girl are you with ...?"

Carrie interrupted Mom midstream, "She's in the living room."

Dad insinuated himself, "Who is this girl—Joe said you had her in your bedroom and that you've been messing around all day?"

They blindsided me. Joe had been devilish with his remarks. They judged me as a fornicator, most likely assuming I had sex with Ra. I was furious. Carrie sat there with her arms folded, without accusation or defense.

I said, "The girl in the other room is my friend, and her name is Ra. I invited her here to watch a movie, and Joe wouldn't surrender the TV, so we went for a walk in the woods!"

Mom shouted me down, "Why did you take her to the woods—why couldn't you watch a show with Joe?"

Here it was again, a festering wound bound up with religion, pushing us further apart.

Dad said, "You need to ask that girl to leave."

By the time I returned to the living room, Ra was moving out the door. I walked her to her car and apologized for the situation. She brushed my worries away with a hug, started her car, and backed out of the driveway. I watched her taillights shrink into the distance until I couldn't see them anymore.

I walked into the house, past the argument in the kitchen, and into my room.

Dad followed me to the door, and accusingly asked, "Who is this girl—did you have intercourse with her?"

Disgusted, I ended the dialogue by stating, "That's your greatest concern about me."

After our day in the woods, I pursued Ra as steadfastly as my parents would have objected. After the incident in the kitchen, I refused any parlay with Mom and Dad and offered Joe no compassion. After school, I spent my time with Toomer and went home only to sleep.

#

Eventually, Ra accepted my invitation to drive her home from school. Ra not riding with Colt was the notification that their relationship was over. I'd given her everything within me and readily devoured any opportunity to be with her. If granted the smallest fraction of time, I was by her side. Our notebooks were now a multivolume set that I kept in my locker. By winter, Ra and I were inseparable.

Shortest Day/Longest Night

A crackling voice coming out of the classroom intercom summoned me to the office. I walked the short distance from my English class to the front desk, where the receptionist notified me of a phone call on hold. I picked up the receiver and depressed the flashing button. Joe was on the line. He informed me he was on his way to pick me up to visit Carrie at Riverview Hospital. The information didn't shock me; it relieved me from returning to class. I hung up the handset, retrieved my notebooks, and sat on the school foyer bench. I stared out the windows and watched the traffic on State Road 13.

Carrie was in the hospital. I wasn't anxious—not because I didn't care deeply about her, but because most every month, for as long as I could remember, I'd had to sit in waiting rooms as Danny or Joe rested on the precipice of eternity. I was seventeen, and for the previous nine years, I'd been in this position innumerable times. For the first couple of years, I didn't have to deal directly with these conflicts as I couldn't wrap my head around what was happening. After I realized the physical threat, I was fearful. I understood my own odds and expected to succumb to the ailment plaguing my siblings. Now, emergency trips to the hospital and dangerous medical procedures bored me. Emotionally painful revelations were such a common occurrence that they no longer affected me. I'd become numb to the constant brushes with death.

Religion didn't help. When the church surrounded our household and prayed for my brother's healing—that failed to materialize—I grew embittered. In the face of the fear and grief that overwhelmed my family, they called for me to have faith while my brothers rotted with brain cancer. The church told me I suffered because I didn't believe God would heal Joe and

Danny. They used the words of Jesus, "If you have faith the size of a grain of mustard seed, miracles will happen."

Clearly, having faith that size wasn't the right recipe for a miracle. After nine years of watching my family battered by disease and feeling the constant challenges of earning salvation, I was now calling bullshit on the entire religious environment. I resented the church's trust in God, their pity, and the continual beam cast on our weakness and infirmity. Faith? Believe in what? I believed in a doctor's ability to mangle my brothers and drug them out of their minds. Pity? If I needed pity, I'd do just as well by asking someone to piss on me. Fuck pity. It's a weak-minded individual's smallest effort to show care or concern and an outward opportunity to claim virtue. I wanted to bomb bridges and separate myself from these rotten ordeals.

Carrie was in the hospital, and Joe was on his way to pick me up? Joe was taking me out of school to transport me to the hospital to be with Carrie. This was most likely ruinous as I was with Carrie a few days before, and she seemed well.

I watched Joe's new silver Firebird round the corner of the parking lot and roll up to the door. The past six months, having no seizures, restored Joe's driving privileges and my freedom from being his chauffeur, cook, and monitor. I didn't hate Joe, but my feelings were close to that point. It was an understatement to say we didn't get along. He embodied everything that confined me. His femininity, religion, and frailty were counter to my spirit. His countless surgeries, bouts of radiation, and chemotherapy treatments caused the skin on one side of his head to settle around his brain, where the doctors permanently removed a hand-sized portion of his skull. Witnessing his wound that never healed made me face my future, and it tormented me. I grudgingly settled down into the vinyl passenger seat and we sped away.

I asked what was wrong with Carrie, and he said, "She's really sick."

"Jesus, Joe—Fucking Christ, what does that mean—why is Carrie in the hospital?"

"Stop cussing, or I'm going to tell Mother!" he screamed.

"Fucking tell her, I don't fucking care."

#

I knew the situation was dreadful when we entered the emergency ward at Riverview and I saw Unck, Aunt Jobee, and a group of people from the church. They sent Joe and me into Carrie's room, where my parents as well as Danny, Laura, and Ted all stood.

Fluid severely swelled Carrie's body, and she was panting. Her face was wet and pale, and her eyes were half open and dim. They guided me to the side of her bed, where I laid my hand on her arm while terror crept along my spine.

She'd been a pillar of strength throughout all the ordeals our family had faced. To see her in this condition was brutality without comparison. I didn't expect to encounter this. It was like a vicious strike to my heart.

I took my hand from her clammy skin, and with tears in my eyes, I said the only thing I could muster, "Carrie, I love you."

Her condition caused her gaze to be locked on the ceiling, but she responded between gasps for air, "I—love—you—Bubby."

I felt shame that my words had caused her to struggle. I stepped back through my family members and went out into the hall. Unck put his arm around my shoulders, and we walked to a small waiting room. I sat down and picked up a magazine, seeking any distraction from this distress. I didn't want to speak to anyone. Besides, who could I talk to without compounding the grief, horror, and sorrow we were all experiencing? Carrie's condition made no sense. My mind swirled in confusion, and I tried to let it blow through me.

Her situation appeared worse than what I'd ever witnessed with Joe or Danny; those moments didn't rise to this level, and I didn't believe she could pull through. Why Carrie? She was twenty-nine with a husband and two young children. She'd even lost her second baby. She withstood the wounds we continually experienced and worked so diligently to repair us, and now she lay wrestling with her own mortality.

I could hear our pastor praying for Carrie, but I knew neither he nor any other savior would pluck her from her fate. Again, the church incensed me by insinuating themselves in our merger with death. I wanted them to leave us alone and not interrupt what remaining time was available.

Dad entered the room. He appeared drawn and damaged, like a prisoner of war paraded in front of a camera. He explained that Carrie had suffered for weeks from flulike symptoms, and her doctor treated her condition with antibiotics. These antibiotics destroyed her bowels' flora and permitted the bacteria in her intestinal tract to migrate internally. She was septic, her kidneys were rapidly failing, and her lungs were filling with fluid, but an experimental treatment was on the way from the West Coast. He'd also contacted the American Red Cross to facilitate Lamech's return from Germany.

The situation painted Dad's face with misery. He'd been in this position twice before, and now a third child was slipping out of his hands.

#

Shortly after nightfall, Carrie lapsed into unconsciousness and they placed her on a ventilator. We took turns standing in her room. We talked to her, but the only response was the ventilator's solo performance. The check valves and pneumatics clicked and pumped in unison. The seal in its cylinder fell as Carrie's swollen chest rose. By morning, we knew she had reached the point of no return, and Ted agreed to remove her from life support. We all gathered around her while the doctor turned off the apparatus that kept Carrie tied to this world. We listened to my sister wheeze and watched her diaphragm collapse.

Fluid gurgled in her throat as she struggled for another wisp of air. I knew what would happen; eventually, one of these efforts would be her last. The room was sick with waiting, hope, prayer, promise, pain, tears, and the sound of Carrie's draw followed by others, each fainter and further apart than the previous. Death lived between each forthcoming depression of her diaphragm and each painful gasp. Being so close to the abyss gave me the feeling that years were peeling off my life. I felt myself and the world around me changing. With each terminal respiration, the light seemed to dim, and I became darker and more feral. As she labored, I wished her to pass and be free. Her ragged breathing continued as a hush fell over us. My father chanced to pray during a pause but silenced himself when she made no further effort. We watched the line on her monitor flatten. Like a trace of morning fog chased by the wind, Carrie's life faded from us.

The motherly hen who sheltered and loved me slipped between the weeds. I recalled the images of the youthful girl I watched breathing in the soft light of dawn and understood with crushing sorrow that I'd never feel the comfort of her presence again. She was with her sisters, and I felt incredibly alone.

#

Carrie's viewing and service, packed with people from across the state, appeared heartwarming but was incredibly sad. She died six months short of her thirtieth birthday and left a young husband with two children, not knowing what to do. Everyone in attendance crumpled under grief for her; she'd been as kind to all of them as she had me, and I'm sure they felt as busted as I did—like your heart and lungs were missing, with nothing but a cold bloody hollow inside your chest. Shortly before the minister took over the podium to speak, my household settled into a pew. Members of my family that had someone leaned into one another with their arms draped over shoulders, and even Joe had one of his ladies to comfort him. Alone, I numbly stared at the floor, until I felt hands slipping around my back and under my arm. I became aware of Ra, fitted in a black dress, wedging herself against me. She'd skipped school to be with me, and I couldn't fathom being more blessed.

We buried Carrie next to her son, Ted Nicholas, in the cemetery along Strawtown Road near Morse Reservoir. I saw the grief in everyone; Mom and Dad caved in, their faces covered in tears, Danny and Joe were weeping, and Lamech stared blankly through the crowd gathered from around the state. I felt like I'd walked down into a body of water with my head below the surface. The lights went out, and I was dark inside. I felt hands patting my back and watched people's mouths move. Numbness settled in and time slipped away.

CHAPTER 7

False Dawn
1989–1992 (17–21 Years Old)

NOT LONG AFTER Carrie's funeral, Ra said she wanted to go to church with me.

I choked and questioned her sanity, "Why would you want to do that?"

"Because I want to!" she shot back.

"Well, I want to be with you, but it ain't much fun there," I affirmed.

By this point, Mom and Dad had begun to accept that I was dating a girl from outside their religion, so they brightened when I informed them that Ra wanted to go to a service with us. The five of us—including Joe—crammed into Dad's sedan. I reveled in being pressed against Ra as we drove to the evening Bible study.

Inside the church, I noticed everyone's eyes on Ra. I monitored her for the smallest reaction throughout the event as the minister shared cringeworthy opinions and verses from the pulpit. Afterward, everyone tried to be as friendly as they had been with Burly years before. I hoped it would have the same effect on Ra, but somehow it didn't. Later that night, when we were alone, I asked her what she thought about the gathering. It dumbfounded me when she said she liked it and wanted to go again.

I didn't know what to think about her interest but welcomed the opportunity to be together without hiding from my parents. She attended the following Sunday services and shocked me when she asked to be baptized. I couldn't make sense of her desire; I'd derided the church since our earliest conversations. Since she was genuinely interested, I couldn't and wouldn't dissuade her; I answered as many of her questions about the Bible and Pentecostalism as possible. She joined the New Converts group, and we went to every service. It was disheartening to watch her enthusiasm progress; the brightest point of light in my life moved closer to everything I'd tried to get away from since I was a boy. After several weeks of attendance, there was an emotional change within her; she was brighter if not bubbly.

When she stopped wearing makeup and short skirts, I was at a loss. I was supportive but felt I was losing her. Eventually she noticed my detachment and questioned me about it. I told her I was happy that she'd discovered a relationship with God but didn't see it as an option for me. I figured I'd cursed him enough to warrant being cut off from what he offered. As was her gift, she had a way of talking me through stressful concerns, and she coaxed me into the possibility of living in God's grace. She was the only light in my life, and I wanted to be wherever she went.

#

We spent more and more time together, sneaking away at every opportunity and rummaging through antique stores. Thoughts of being apart and furthering our education in different states seemed like a path to avoid. The day we graduated from high school, I gave her a promise ring and we agreed to marry.

Our summer was sweet and unencumbered with any worry. On the Fourth of July, I offered her an engagement ring and she accepted my proposal. We planned a two-year courtship involving everything a couple might need to be successful, ranging from counseling and wedding showers to mundane tasks like sourcing kitchen sundries and lawn equipment.

Our engagement didn't settle well with either set of parents. Mom and Dad were crestfallen over my decision to reject an invitation from Columbia College of the Arts in Chicago. Ra's stepfather believed our union would be more akin to World War III.

Not long after my eighteenth birthday, Ra and I bought a factory home in the Meadowbrook addition of Anderson and each evening and weekend, we worked on fixing its failures. Fifty years of paint sealed the windows and we spent two weeks freeing them from it so they would open. The living-room ceiling looked like a jigsaw puzzle with a couple of pieces missing, so we knocked it down and installed new drywall and a fresh topcoat of plaster. We wallpapered our bedroom and refit the plastic tiles on the kitchen walls. Ra uprooted all the weeds and vines that covered the fence encircling our extra lot, and Dad helped me upright and brace the twisting detached garage. The front sidewalk flooded when it rained, so I sledgehammered it to rubble and laid reclaimed brick in a herringbone pattern. Each day, after ten hours at the shop, I had dinner with my parents in Anderson and drove to Lapel to pick up Ra. From there, we went to our little home, worked until midnight, and then I drove her back to Lapel before coasting to Lone Oak to sleep for a few moments. This schedule ground me down until one autumn night, after dropping Ra off at her house, I fell asleep while driving, crossed the center lane, and blasted into a telephone pole. I was uninjured, but this event pressed us to advance our wedding date to the coming winter.

#

In August, Unck called to inform me that Mrs. Cooper could no longer care for Luther and transferred him to a nursing home. When I received the news, I feared losing my friends. I asked Ra if she'd be interested in visiting the Coopers, and she was.

When we arrived on Josephine Street, the first thing I noticed was Mrs. Cooper working in her garden. I approached the property, calling her name, and she faced me in the same fashion as she always had but bowed more by time. She gazed at me over her battered glasses instead of through them and seemed confused, as if she didn't recognize me.

I realized I'd changed tremendously in the twelve years I'd been away, so I introduced myself. Wrinkles formed between her eyes like she couldn't see me. I shared my name again, and she shook her head, confirming her lack of knowledge. It felt like a rope was slipping between my hands, so I laid bare all the moments I could remember, pleading for their existence and hoping that something I said could kindle a fire in her mind, but the only thing I grasped was that I was now a stranger to her. To my great sadness, Lola could not tie a memory to my name, face, or events on Josephine Street.

After a brief silence, she chuckled, kindly, apologized for her lack of recall, turned away, and quietly shuffled into the ordered rows of vegetables until I could no longer see her. I knew I would never see her again.

Ra and I walked back to our car. I couldn't find words to express my loss. I felt like another part of me was gone forever.

#

In January 1991, two weeks before our wedding, Danny blacked out from a seizure while at work. From Universal Tool, the ambulance transferred him to IU Hospital, where the radiology department found a blood clot filling the space from the removal of his brain tumor. The surgical staff performed emergency surgery, but it seemed to cripple him more than it helped. He'd planned to be an usher in our wedding but gracefully declined.

#

The day of our wedding, January 19, 1991, the sky was gray with a threat of snow. We'd spent the past six months preparing invitations and decorations for the ceremony. It was like a dream, watching the bridesmaids in hunter-green velvet carrying candles down the darkened aisle. Ra's entrance brought tears to my eyes; she was stunning in her satin and embroidered gown.

As Ra passed the pews occupied by friends and family, I couldn't help but notice Danny's frail body with a wet incision twisting around his scalp and the whites of his eyes filled with clots of blood from the surgery. And I was reminded of Carrie's absence, but as quickly as that thought came, I put it out of my mind. It was so easy to ignore terrible things when I was with Ra. She made me feel alive when every other thing didn't. If life were a gemstone, she was the facet that caught the sun. She was Carrie in the dim light of dawn, Brinson in the

Coopers' yard, the warmth in Mamaw's kitchen, the mist that hung above fields, the sunset in front of us, and the whisper of rain on water. She was starlight and the sound of tree peepers at night, and I was the darkness surrounding her.

#

A few weeks after our wedding, Danny's CT scan revealed recent tumor growth filling the void from his first surgery. The rapidly growing cancer and his impaired health left no option for further treatment. He and Laura planned what they wanted to do before he couldn't do anything more. In March, they traveled with their daughter to Disney World, and on returning, Danny entered home hospice. He quickly withered and was often lost in confusion. The evening of April 5, he closed his eyes to sleep and didn't wake the next morning. An ambulance took him to IU Medical Center, where the staff settled him in a room. He remained unresponsive and three days later, on April 8, 1991, his labored breathing ceased.

For his burial, we carried Danny to Mechanicsburg, Indiana. The decision not to bury him in the Gadd family plot bothered me, but Carrie wasn't there either. I thought the town's name was fitting; Danny always seemed to have a wrench in his hands. When we were boys, he borrowed tools from Dad's toolbox and built us bicycles from scrap parts. As a teen, he tinkered with Cox engines and cars and used a fistful of pencils to improve Kenny Keenhound's behavior. He followed Dad into the tool and die trade and wrenched on machines until his body failed him. On this day, his hands were useless, empty, cold, and crossed on his abdomen. He couldn't work anymore, and there wasn't anyone to repair us.

Danny was twenty-nine when he died. He was a powerful figurehead in my life, and his passing was like having something forcibly extracted from my person. Danny was rakish, foolhardy, and never gave a damn; he was everything the rest of us never needed to be because he'd always been there. He fought brain cancer and all that it brought for a third of his existence. It relieved me that he couldn't suffer anymore, but the suffering didn't go into the ground with him; it took up residence in all of us.

Joe assessed his sorrow and the situation by coldly stating, "I thought I'd die before Danny."

#

Little more than two years divided the deaths of Carrie and Danny. I refused to think about it in any way other than acknowledging that I missed them. I went through the motions of working, going to church, and keeping a home. Every day appeared overcast, as if a weather front had settled in and blocked the sun. Nights seemed unusually dark, and artificial lighting didn't help. Everything looked out of focus, like trying to see through a fog. My three-month marriage was suffering, the pastor at Temple Mount removed me from participating in worship activities, and work took more from me than I could trade.

Although I was nineteen, my boyhood fears returned; I worried over headaches, twitches in my eye, and muscle spasms. I felt weak, ineffectual, and rudderless. I wanted to be happy and I thought I should be. Ra and I were married and starting a new life with the world at our feet, but holding that up against Danny's passing was like trying to kindle a fire in a rain-laden wind.

I felt broken, but I didn't voice what I was feeling. I didn't know that I could or should. Hell, we'd all gone through this before. We'd all struggled inwardly with Joe and Danny slowly dying. Mom and Dad had buried Garnna, Shelam, Carrie, and Danny, refusing to complain or publicly express any significant discomfort or grief. As glorious examples of courage, they bore their burdens stoically year after year, and the people they encountered were none the wiser. I could do the same; I'd done it before and could do it again. I just needed to toughen up, keep my mouth shut, and repress all the dread. If I gave myself a little time—maybe a few weeks or months—it would all be normal.

Halocline

Joe's MRI in January 1992 called the faith proclaimed by the church into question. It seemed the more they prayed, the faster his tumor grew. The more they preached about belief in Jesus's miracle-working powers, the weaker he became. Joe's health was like a candle in the wind, and it was withering day by day. He knew there wouldn't be any more surgeries, and he understood—from Danny's example—how he would pass. He accepted it with grace, and his anger faded. It was sad to see him this way; his spunk and characteristic grit dissolved. He didn't lose his usual sass but didn't apply it with relish.

At this time, it seemed cruelty touched every moment. The church ascribed these circumstances to the work of Satan and original sin. I wasn't confident or arrogant enough to place weight on either, but it did feel like we were all cursed. When I lined up all the events, they appeared connected—as if my family's roots fed from some poisoned aquifer. I saw Carrie drowning on her deathbed. I heard Danny's scream for help at his first seizure. I remembered the day after Joe's eighteenth birthday and the feeling of something moving underground. I pondered Dad's dream and the name it gave me. I felt Shelam dying in Padanaram and wondered about Garnna, taken by meningitis. I thought of all these things conspiring against us, repeatedly, trying to find a reason, and it turned my insides black.

#

Lamech and Tonya returned to the States, and he left the service. Shortly after, they divorced. It was an enormous blow to Mom and Dad; they'd invested a substantial number of prayers and a trove of energy in supporting the union. This event, paired with the loss of life, was hurtful, like a failed crop at harvest.

#

In February, Ra told me she was pregnant. It was exciting and terrifying news. During our engagement, we talked about having a large brood of sons and daughters. A year before, it was fun making plans and dreaming about all sorts of things that make you glow inside. Now, under the shadow of the dead and dying, and the potential of carrying a curse, the thought of being a father wasn't a crown I expected to wear.

I thought of Dad after Garnna's death. Losing an infant—no one willingly thinks of that; it's not uncommon, but it's not something you think will happen to you. It happened to Dad, but after spawning three more healthy kids, it probably seemed like a fluke—until Shelam died. By the time they diagnosed Joe and Danny with the same kind of tumor that Shelam had, there was a pattern. When Carrie perished unexpectedly, the writing was on the wall. I had no reason to expect I'd dodged the bullet. I could fall shaking at any minute and leave a wife and baby to watch me slowly die. Worst of all, I likely had passed whatever my family had on to my offspring. I witnessed the joy in Ra's eyes, and I envisioned them filled with tears over a dying child. Being terrified made me feel like a shitbag; Dad was out in the middle of a storm, and I ached at the threat of rain. I felt poisoned and guilty and established a pact with myself to limit any further damage.

#

Ra's pregnancy wasn't easy; various conditions forced her to visit the emergency pavilion at Riverview Hospital or rest in bed for weeks at a time. The first event was a blood-soaked, high-speed run to Noblesville. Our critical-care nurse informed us that Ra had most likely miscarried. I held Ra as she shuddered and cried, but just after midnight, the ultrasound technician found a heartbeat and a properly formed fetal pole. Next to this proof of life was a disintegrating fraternal twin.

#

On August 11, 1992, Ra's contractions, coupled with amniotic fluid, caused us to rush to the hospital. They admitted Ra to the maternity ward and family members set up camp in the waiting room. Her labor continued through the night and into the morning. She worried about our baby's lack of movement and mentioned it to the nurses, but they brushed off her concerns. That afternoon, a nurse conducting her rounds checked Ra's monitor; panic-stricken, she dove across Ra to hit the intercom and screamed for help. Within seconds, nurses flooded into our space. I jumped back to make way as they went to work prepping Ra for an emergency cesarean section. In less than a minute, they wheeled her into the surgery ward. All I could do was follow the procession, while Ra cried.

As they told me to take a seat next to the door, I felt a switch click within me. My mind went quiet, expecting another failure of life. I slipped into a semicatatonic state—familiar in these situations—and thumbed through an available magazine while thinking of Carrie's Ted Nicholas, stillborn though fully developed. I saw his pale body in his miniature coffin. I thought I was losing my child, wife, or both.

Within a few minutes, the door swung open and a nurse shoved a gown and face mask at me, telling me to follow her. We walked briskly down the hall and into a surgery bay. I didn't expect good fortune and didn't think to ask any questions. As we rounded the corner, I saw nurses tending to a squirming newborn child, and on my right, I saw Ra being sutured from her surgery. A nurse swaddled the infant in a blanket, brought it to me, and told me that everything was fine.

She pressed the baby against my chest and said, "This is your daughter!"

I cradled the bundle in my arms and held her to my cheek as tears filled my eyes. She cried to the world with a slight chattering sound that reminded me of a chipmunk. I paced back and forth, staring at her little red face and dark hair until the nurses ushered me into the nursery. The doctor entered and informed me that Ra was just fine; the cause of the problem was the umbilical cord wrapped around our infant so many times that she couldn't descend and went into distress. She pointed to the viewing window and said, "Daddy, you've got some people that want to see that baby!"

I turned to see our parents and Ra's sisters giddy with joy. It felt like my insides were on fire as I held her to the window for them to see. I felt joy like I hadn't in such a long time; it was like being in Unck's airplane, just after leaving the ground.

Ra chose to call our child Morgan Ra, and that's what she was, our morning sun. After a couple of days, we packed her into our car and drove to our tiny house in Anderson. She was a pleasure! We dropped into a perfect routine. On returning from work, I'd feed and cradle her on the couch and then would put her in her bassinet just after midnight. When my alarm went off at 4:00 a.m., I'd hold her for a bit before laying her in bed with Ra.

#

By November, Joe's physical and cognitive abilities declined. The steroids he took to prevent brain swelling caused an incredible amount of weight gain. Over the summer, after his last MRI, he stopped wearing the hairpiece that Mom and Dad had custom-manufactured for him, and it sat on its foam block near his bed. The fluid filling the once sunken wound over his right brow gave the impression his skull wasn't disfigured. His eyes were dull and expressionless, and the tumor activity and medication slurred his speech. Ra, with Morgan and other family friends, stayed with Joe during odd hours. They served him tea and carried on with him—wherever his mind went. He was occasionally his sassy self, like a fish coming to the surface of an inky pool.

December was wet and gray, and we knew Joe was near his end. Dad rented a hospital bed, erected it in my old bedroom, and installed a recliner. A hospice nurse visited Joe to check his vital signs and help him with his showers. Mom informed as many of Joe's friends that she could find that he was passing. They drove from all over the state to visit and whisper words to him as he slept. All of his ladies from various churches filled his room. They held his delicate hand and caressed his arm, crying and wishing him well. They thanked him for being who he was. They reminded him of the things he'd made for them over the years, and how much they cherished his friendship. They recounted the moments he'd teased them into being better people and told him he was the strongest person they'd ever known. They pulled crumpled tissues from their purses to dab at tiny tears rolling down their cheeks.

They kissed his forehead, patted his cheek, and whispered, "Goodbye, Joey."

#

On December 15, Joe—spurred to consciousness by his bath—casually informed the hospice nurse, "I'm going home."

Later that evening, as Mom tucked him into bed, he spoke again, "I'm going home."

He drifted into sleep, and his respiration was shallow and irregular.

As night watch, I was alone with him and knew it was our time to part. My tears didn't come to me as they did with Carrie and Danny. I thought of how the ground between Joe and me was uneven and hard to navigate, and how we'd invariably riled each other. I considered how everybody seemed to love him but me, and I felt shame. I felt I should love him but couldn't find that feeling within me. Maybe we'd been too long and too close to the fire. I'd been his sitter, chauffeur, subject of taunts, caterer, and escort. For ten years, the illness of Joe Gadd touched—if not dominated—everything. I'd always been in its gaze and couldn't hide from it even when I tried. It terrorized me throughout the day and kept me awake at night. It forced me to constantly be on guard. It twisted me to do shameful things and darkened my pride. It took from everyone; there wasn't a peaceful shred that it didn't harbor for itself. I knew it wasn't Joe that warred against me, but I saw him in the mirror each time I passed one. He was all I didn't want to be and everything I expected to become. He, and all that he endured, shaped every little and large thing in my life.

I was sorry for all that had happened to him. I looked back on all my cruelties toward him and thought of him as a boy, making cornhusk dolls at the edge of a field in the sunlight of summer. I recognized him as the gentle older brother who liked to carry me on his shoulders around the house in Martinsville. I saw him as the young man that did everything he said he would. I remembered him as the only person I'd ever known who struggled so hard for so long and remained unbowed. I laid my hand on his frail wrist, looked over his swollen scar to his freckled and pockmarked face, and told him I loved him. Rightly so, there would be no response.

In the morning hours of December 16, 1992, the life within Joseph Michael Gadd took flight.

#

Thanks to Joe's many friends and acquaintances, his wake and two funeral services were as massive and as beautiful as he would have demanded. Multiple musicians played and sang his favorite songs. Several people spoke about his fine qualities and how they inspired them. The pastor delivered a message on Joe's tribulations and chanced to imagine that he was now dancing, free of all ailments, with his departed brother and sisters. He said Joe was victorious over death and the grave, and that one day we would all see him again. The procession to his graveside was more than three miles long.

In the cold rain, we laid him between Garnna and Shelam, under the bare oaks of South Park Cemetery in Martinsville.

#

Joe's passing settled on us quietly. There was the sadness that comes with losing anyone, but there was a peacefulness to it, a reverent thankfulness for not being held to witness the suffering of one of our own. We were wrung out and riddled with a multitude of damages we'd never had thought or time to address. Like mariners who'd passed through a typhoon, we'd made landfall and were crawling along the shore, not yet aware that we were alive. It cratered my insides, and again I was numb to everything else.

The week before Christmas, Ra suggested that we set up the family Christmas tree for Mom and Dad and try to make this holiday as pleasant as possible. They accepted her sentiment. Four days after Joe's funeral, we bundled Morgan into the car and drove to their house.

Along the way, Ra talked about the prospect of living a life without someone perishing and wondered what that might be like for us. I was tired from my day at the tool shop but looked forward to a long Christmas weekend. She knew I was down, and she said all the right words that brought me up. I hadn't thought my life could be any different. I never considered imagining what my world could be like without Danny or Joe slowly dying, but it settled in as we pulled up to the house.

We found Mom preparing a pot of potato soup and Dad with all the boxes of Christmas decorations stacked in the living room. After dinner, we unpacked everything Joe had stored the year before. We assembled his artificial tree from Toles Flowers and wrapped it with lights, heirloom ornaments, and Joe's most prized trinkets. We played Joe's gospel Christmas albums and recalled our favorite memories of him.

CHAPTER 8

Killing Owls
1993–1996 (21–25 Years Old)

IN LATE JANUARY, Ra noticed Morgan holding her breath while her torso seemed to seize in contractions. Morgan was four months old and was born with hemangiomas on her nose and hip. Icy fear gripped us, and we scheduled an electroencephalogram (EEG) at Riley Hospital for Children (IU) in Indianapolis.

To say it was unnerving to need to take Morgan to IU Medical Center is an understatement. As we walked across the campus, I couldn't swallow or catch my breath. My ears were ringing, and it felt like there were hornets in my brain. I'd spent over ten years following my brothers in and out of there as it disfigured them and they slowly died. I had the brief lives and brutal deaths of Garnna and Shelam on my mind.

We checked in and the nurse directed us to an older wing of the hospital, where we found our intake room. After a few minutes, the specialist entered and did a cursory exam of Morgan. He asked about family history and paused when Ra brought up my recent past. I told him about Joe, Danny, and Shelam but didn't mention Carrie or Garnna. He said that an EEG might find something and left the room. A team of nurses came in and applied padded sensors to Morgan's head and torso. They conducted the test and then suggested we go to the cafeteria for lunch while the doctor looked over the results.

#

The cafeteria hadn't changed since Danny's last surgery. The only open seats we found were in the same enclave where I heard the results of Joe's first surgery.

I stirred the black beans with rice on my plate while Ra fed Morgan. My insides were turning over. We avoided the subject of why we were there, but commented on the cardinals outside the window and the Mardi Gras parade on the TV.

#

At 1:00, we made our way back to our room and waited for the doctor to return. Within a few minutes, he entered and told us that something was on the EEG but felt it didn't warrant further investigation. He prescribed phenobarbital and a monitor to track Morgan's heart rate and respiration. He curtly suggested that she had epilepsy. We pressed him for a thorough assessment, and he brushed off what he found as a misfire. Saying that "the phenobarbital will take care of it," he ushered us out of the room.

I fumed and gnashed my teeth on the way to the parking garage. The doctor's cursory investigation upset me; everything within me screamed against giving Morgan barbiturates.

#

As directed, we rented the monitor for Morgan and pasted its leads to her torso for the next few months. Its alarm sounded when her respiration dropped below a safe threshold, occasionally while napping and a few times each night. Not wanting to be the bearers of fearful news after Joe's burial, we decided not to tell Mom or Dad about the situation.

As our plight stretched into summer, we couldn't hold the fear at bay and Ra finally spoke with Mom. Mom contacted one of Joe's physicians and he scheduled an MRI for Morgan. The results revealed a suspicious area in her brain that he determined to be a mass of blood vessels. He noted the hemangiomas on Morgan's hip and nose and suggested it was most likely the same thing. He was concerned that it was an issue but believed it would subside as she grew. He asked us to keep her on the monitor but didn't see any reason to prescribe medication. By the end of the year, Morgan's symptoms faded along with her birthmarks.

#

In deep winter, my relationship with the church and religion reached a terminal point. There was an admonition to pursue continual spiritual growth, but the more I sought it, the more there seemed to be a ceiling. I'd unwillingly and willfully tried to be Christlike for almost twenty years and couldn't honestly say that I was anywhere near the goalpost. Truthfully accounting, I'd studied the King James Bible cover to cover multiple times and had sat through teachings and services on more occasions than I could count. I'd meditated, prayed, and requested guidance on my spiritual path, but it felt like I was trying to grow something in barren ground.

Ra and I thought of attending another church, hoping it might help. We reached out to a neighboring parish in our fellowship, and the minister welcomed us but wanted to make sure our current pastor was in line with the move. When we sought an agreement, our pastor seemed insulted and suggested, in several ways, that leaving Temple Mount for a different congregation would be detrimental to our souls. His language sounded so counter to his familiar demeanor and sermons that it was like taking a punch to the forehead. Ra and I tried to ignore our feelings. We wanted to do the right thing and not endanger ourselves with Christ. We stayed on and struggled to fix ourselves.

By spring, we were in the same position and, again, I reached out to the church in Noblesville. When I spoke with the pastor who had welcomed us in the winter, he asked us not to join his congregation as ours informed him we were troublemakers. Although this incident was crushing, Ra and I maintained our dedication and attendance.

After a few more months of services, I had an overwhelming feeling of completeness. In the middle of a Wednesday-night Bible study, I realized that I had nothing more to learn from studying the Bible and attending services. I'd experienced so many sermons and teachings I could finish any new one by rote within the first few sentences. There wasn't anything left to sacrifice or anything of value to better my spirit. I wasn't scared, hurt, disappointed, or left questioning; I drifted in limbo.

#

After another day at the tool shop, Ra met me at the door with a pack of cassette tapes and implored me to listen to them. I waved her off and went to take a shower.

She followed me, holding the recordings in front of her, and exclaimed, "We're in a cult, and we've got to get out of there!"

I immediately pictured Jim Jones and bloated corpses in a jungle village. "What do you mean, we're in a cult?"

She responded with her account of listening to a weeklong Christian radio program about religious cults and toxic faith. It affected her so powerfully that she called into the show for a transcript and a set of tapes. I didn't know what to think about her accusation and refused to listen to the program. She countered my response by shoving the first tape into our stereo and turned up the volume loud enough to penetrate the walls of our 400-square-foot home. I couldn't get away from it, but I wasn't going to leave the house. She repeated her actions, every evening, for the following few weeks.

A cult? My family wasn't in a cult. I hadn't been in a cult since I was four! Mamaw, Unck, Joe, Carrie, and Mom and Dad wouldn't be in a cult. The idea of accusing our church of being a cult was tantamount to an unpardonable sin. The thought of my family's religion being false felt convicting.

Each night, she hit me with those tapes like she was trying to break a criminal suspect. After the first few sessions, I opened my ears to the personal accounts of victims and methodologies of predators preying on undeveloped minds. As I allowed myself to question, it wasn't difficult to visualize the patterns. Eventually, I could draw a line between every action I'd witnessed and every moment I'd bent myself to someone's will. I could see where they'd groomed me to accept everything without question. Now, I had question after question. I couldn't lie to myself about it, and I couldn't lie to Ra.

The program offered a list of resources and connections to independent psychologists and counselors in various regions. We found a counselor in Indianapolis and secretly scheduled our first meeting on a Tuesday evening so we wouldn't miss Wednesday's Bible study.

#

Our counselor, Henry Thompson, was a retired Army chaplain who'd spent most of his private practice helping victims of abuse and trauma. We devoted two evenings each week for the remainder of the summer and into September to our counseling sessions, unpacking our hearts and minds with Henry. To say it was challenging and stressful doesn't fully describe what we went through. We dealt with seemingly insurmountable issues; failed relationships, tragedy, abuse, grief, and cult activity are generic labels for aggregations of unpackaged damages and agreements with oneself. Unfortunately, these aren't things that, once talked about, fade away. Mostly, it's a matter of consistently and continually pulling at the splinters; just when you think you've dug the last of it out, you'll run across something that snags another one. We learned how to examine our feelings and thoughts and assess the filters through which we viewed our world. After we rounded some sharp corners on ourselves and our relationship, we burrowed into our connections with authority, religion, spiritualism, hierarchies, and why humans subjugate and control other people.

#

In mid-September, Ra and I found the understanding and ability to admit that our religious beliefs and environment were coercive, abusive, and isolating. We knew acutely that the situation was toxic. We couldn't stay where we were but giving up the congregation meant leaving Mom and Dad and friends of

THE BIRD'S ROAD		199

many years; every way we looked at it was hurtful. We didn't take this lightly; on our exit, we realized they would cast aspersions against us, and they would admonish those that stayed to cease fellowship with us. We'd be thought of as something less if not far worse than any of them. They'd call us backsliders and consider us cut off from God.

We wanted to be upright in our departure, so we scheduled an appointment to inform the senior pastor. On the way home from the tool shop a few days before our session, I told Dad about what transpired, our counseling, and our intended move away from the church. He took it sorely but offered to join us at our meeting.

After all the grievous things I'd been part of, the thought of this meeting surprised me by riddling me with anxiety. I'd never stood up for myself; I'd always been like water and found paths over, under, or around obstructions. This was the first occasion I'd squared with something, and that object was more than an acquaintance, it was an extended family. I wasn't angry, and I carried no malice toward the church. I'd learned a lot there, and I was thankful. I knew I'd miss my old fishing buddies and the ladies who'd been sweet to my household, but it was beyond time for us to get away and find a spiritual environment that fit what we needed.

My parents met us at Temple Mount. We entered the business wing and made our way to the pastor's office, where he, his wife, son, and daughter-in-law were seated. We closed the door behind us and sat in opposing chairs. The pastor and his family seemed surprised to see Mom and Dad. The pastor looked past me and asked my parents why they were there. I responded that Ra and I had come to let them know we were leaving the church. From there, the meeting went south, and toward the end, it turned malicious. It didn't seem they were as concerned about Ra and me joining another parish as they were with losing my parents. Ultimately, they tried to drive a wedge between us by insinuating that we didn't want Mom and Dad involved in Morgan's upbringing. At that moment, it felt like a diamond pierced my mind and froze the room in position. I suddenly understood every faint outline of mental and emotional posturing in the place. For the first time in my life, I felt a new power inside of me, and realized that my mouth was moving with a voice I didn't recognize.

I'd never spoken with authority to authority; clearly and soundly, I called out the revelation illuminated in my heart, "You people are trying to separate me from my family, and it is evil!"

The room fell silent. I felt the fear within the pastor and his family. It wasn't fear of me or what I said, but fear of losing my parents. They'd called Mom and Dad, "Pillars of the Church." They knew that if my parents left the congregation, there would be questions they couldn't answer, and the fallout could cause more members to leave. A mass exodus would cascade into a substantial financial impact.

I'd never expected my parents to leave with us, and it wasn't something that I would ask of them. I wasn't interested in any squabble; I came to offer my resignation in as dignified a manner as I thought I should. After I spoke my assessment, the meeting wrapped up quickly, and the four of us left. It was disappointing to have gone where we had with the church and trusted them for so long, only to find we didn't mean much to them. The course of the session and their actions struck Ra and me as callous, but more important, the positive change of direction in our lives came as a relief.

Weeks later, Dad informed me that they would stay with the congregation; he feared a departure might shake others' faith in God. He asked if we'd discovered another church, and I told him we hadn't. His advice was to make sure I paid my tithes and offerings when I found a place of worship.

Sadly, everything transpired just as Henry predicted.

#

For most of the following year, we maintained our counseling with Henry. The time and education we received from him were the most valuable resources Ra and I had ever encountered. Not long after we ended our sessions, his practice called to tell us that he'd experienced a severe stroke. The event destroyed his memory and most of his mental faculties. The end of his work was a terrible loss to the world.

#

In the months following Joe's death, Mom and Dad resigned themselves to where they'd been and how their world had changed. They continued working and spent their weekends in a small camper on a lake in Brazil, Indiana. For the first time in their lives, they didn't have anyone to care for but themselves. It may have been age, but it seemed like all their emotional damages were surfacing and manifesting as health issues. Mom required knee surgery and received a diagnosis of fibromyalgia. Dad was in and out of the hospital a few times; he detached his bicep while moving machinery at the tool shop and was diagnosed with gallstones. In the summer of 1994, he experienced severe headaches and abused acetaminophen to treat them.

I'd taken a new job at a commercial sign company in Indianapolis. I was excited to be out of Universal Tool and using my abilities in a trade that matched my talents. Conveniently, I worked directly across the interstate from Universal Tool, but Dad and I stopped sharing a ride as our work hours were different.

#

A few weeks before Thanksgiving, Dad wanted to change the fixtures in Lone Oak's full bath, so I showed up Saturday morning to tackle the task. Lamech was also there to help, and Dad gave us some instructions and a box with a new faucet. He put on his Sperry's, told us he needed to get more parts to finish the plumbing, and left in his station wagon. Lamech and I went to work dismantling the shower face.

After more than a few hours, we remarked that Dad was gone longer than expected. Mom called from her work to check on our progress, and Lamech complained about Dad's absence.

Another half hour passed before Dad came home. He entered the house, saying nothing to us, and stumbled into the living room. We followed him and saw him fall into his chair, hold his head in his palms, rock back and forth, and weep. The sight paralyzed me. I didn't know what to say or do, so I escaped to the bathroom to mend a leak. I lacked thought and fumbled with tools as Lamech ran to the kitchen and called Mom. I heard him recounting Dad's behavior, and I felt nauseous and confused. I knew something was dreadfully wrong, but all I could focus on was stopping leaks.

I felt cowardly as I listened to Lamech trying to reason with Dad. Above Lamech's voice, I could hear Dad moaning and speaking gibberish. I crept back to the living room and saw Lamech kneeling next to him, hoping to calm him, but he was inconsolable. Then, I noticed that Dad was wearing two different shoes.

Mom eventually arrived. She got through to Dad, coaxed him into her car, and drove him to the emergency room at Riverview Hospital. Lamech and I stayed at Lone Oak and finished the plumbing repairs in silence, waiting for information.

#

After sedation and a CT scan, they transferred Dad to IU Hospital. The staff ushered Mom into a room and confirmed that Dad had what appeared to be a brain tumor and that only surgery could relieve his symptoms.

Mom returned to Lone Oak and wept the news to us. I felt the bottom drop out of my soul. A feral growl rolled within me. All I could think was, "How and why?" I raged at the prognosis and spat at the minutiae of medical jargon. My mind whirled, both accepting and rejecting facts. Why? Why now? Why Dad? Wasn't everyone else enough? God damn! How? What now? What the fuck? Hasn't enough been taken from us? Do we owe more? Weren't Garnna and Shelam and Carrie and Danny and Joe enough? Do you want more? Fuck this and fuck everything! There is no God, and there is no good! There is no Jesus or any other protector! It's all a goddamn fucking lie, and it always was! Fuck it all!

We all caved inside. There is no word for what we felt. You could dig through any thesaurus and not come close to describing what churned within us.

How did it happen? Why the cruel joke? Why, less than a year after Joe's passing, did the cancer show in Dad? Why did it hit him at an advanced age and not as a child? Was it his aggregated wishes to take the years of pain from his children? Did it finally come home to roost like the vultures in the trees outside Padanaram? It was all just sickening, and denial wasn't an option.

#

Dad held strong through his surgery, and like Danny and Joe, he rebounded quickly. He underwent radiation and chemotherapy treatment. His immobility provoked him to research the cancers of Shelam, Joe, and Danny. His queries illuminated the fact that many of his direct relatives had died of breast, prostate, colon, or ovarian cancers. In his Franklin Planner, he'd drawn a family tree with names and cancer cases. Before his parents' union, there were no notable instances of the disease on his father's side; his mother must have been the source.

At IU Medical Center, he chanced to meet a doctor involved in genetic research. Based on our family history and Dad's suspicions, she suggested investigating tissue stored from Danny and Joe and also Dad's blood. He agreed, and within a few months, he received the results of the test. The report stated in part:

> Dear Mr. and Mrs. Gadd,
>
> As you will recall, we reviewed Li-Fraumeni syndrome in that it is a familial cancer syndrome with multiple different types of tumors being expressed in families which can include brain tumors, leukemia, sarcomas, and adrenal cortical tumors.
>
> The gene, p53, is known as a tumor suppressor gene. This class of gene works as "the brakes of a car" and slows down the cell cycle allowing for repair or selected destruction of abnormal cells. In order for tumors to develop, both copies of this gene must be mutated; therefore, you inherit one mutated copy in all the cells of your body and the second gene is mutated in the brain tissue giving rise to brain tumors.

We discussed your family pedigree, with your sister with bilateral lung cancer, another sister with ovarian cancer and possibly your brother with colon cancer [who] may have inherited this same mutation. We discussed autosomal dominant inheritance which means that you have a 50% chance of passing on the gene mutation to each of your children; therefore, most likely, your three children who developed brain cancer also had this mutation.

There is nothing you did or didn't do to cause a mutation in yourself or pass this on to your children. As you have long suspected this is an inherited condition that most likely originated with your mother and was passed on to you and then to your children.

In Dad's sitting room, from his chair, he shared the report with me. As he read the words, he rubbed the palm of his unoccupied hand across the white stubble of his shaved head, while tears pooled in his eyes. Despite the final lines of the report, he felt implicated in our misery and expressed anguish as the cause for the suffering of Shelam, Joe, and Danny. He recognized the twenty-two years of stress, worry, work, and pain compressed onto an 8.5" x 11" piece of trifolded paper, and absorbed it like a shotgun blast to his chest.

#

Eventually, Dad returned to Universal Tool on a shortened workday. With his new schedule, I could drive him to and from work each day. We both knew his future would be a struggle, and it was a pleasure to pick him up each morning and talk on the way. The role reversal was stimulating to both of us; I had a fresh chance to ask questions, and he relished the opportunity to share. I asked him about his father and mother and all the minuscule details of living in Bucktown. He shared his experiences of surviving alone and how he managed not to starve or freeze. He divulged his feelings on wanting to make a family as his twelve-year-old self envisioned it. I asked about his prior experiences with religion. He admitted that his early forays into churches were to feed himself on Sundays, but they opened doors for employment and principled individuals' generosity. He confided in me that he heard God's voice as a boy and couldn't discount it. He told me how he'd always felt indebted to the people around Morgan County who had helped him stay alive. That's why we'd spent so many weekends fixing equipment and dilapidated houses, cleaning sheds, and delivering supplies when we lived on Josephine Street. He laughed about us fishing at Larry Hess's fish hatchery, hunting for mushrooms, berries, and persimmons; he'd made it an adventure because he couldn't afford to sustain us all on groceries. I questioned his involvement with Jim Jones and David. He said that it just felt right; he wanted to experience God's mystery, and they offered it in those environments unlike in the traditional churches he attended. He spoke of the feeling that God had a hand in his life and directed his path. He reiterated that God foretold my existence and named me before birth.

Joking, I asked him why he gave me such a shitty name, and he smacked me in the ribs, saying, "That's for you to find out!"

I asked about his experiences with past-life regression, and he shared that he could never reach a hypnotic state that allowed him to see his past but mentioned that Mom's experience took her to a past life where she had given birth near an ocean to the rhythm of the waves.

Each morning provided a new topic that filled the half-hour drive to Universal Tool. I'd let him out in the office parking lot and watch him stumble every fifth step until he made it inside the building. I knew better than to try to help him; he wouldn't have accepted it.

#

Through the following summer, Dad recovered just as well as Joe and Danny ever did, but without the strength that youth gives. His hair returned but was whiter. He was almost as agile as before but lost all the muscle he'd carried since I'd known him. He was fit enough to operate a vehicle and work his regular hours again. He decided to drive himself back and forth to the tool shop, and I missed our conversations.

#

When crime escalated around our little home in Meadowbrook, Ra and I sold out and moved into a partially renovated farmhouse on Ford Street in Lapel. Ra enrolled at Anderson University, and I undertook the finishing of our new residence. It was a lot of fun raising Morgan in our old haunts, and rebuilding our new place was rewarding.

#

Over the sale of a vintage sign, we met Richard (Dick) Crenshaw. He'd recently purchased Bonge's Tavern in Perkinsville and spent most of his days avoiding its restoration. He threatened to finish it by the autumn, but he bandied that idea around like Mel Fisher's daily affirmation to find the Nuestra Señora de Atocha's sunken wreck.

Dick was a rare breed of human. Where most men value wealth, renown, and title, he passionately involved himself in discovering the historical gems, in every nook and cranny, that Indiana offered. He knew the most scenic paths to mom-and-pop hamburger stands, notorious place markers, and defunct nunneries like the back of his hand. Ra, Morgan, and I skipped our daily duties at least once a week to run with him on adventures to source material for his tavern.

I'd never met anyone like Crenshaw; he seemed to be pieced together from uncles and best friends. From him, I learned how to be comfortable with strangers and to carry on a conversation. He spurred curiosity and opened my mind to see the world in a fresh light. With a distinct ability to perceive people's fears and social inadequacies, Richard was quick in his comedy to ease them into comfort with themselves. Over dinner and a few drinks, he could tease out someone's darkest moments and make them feel it was okay to be alive. In a way, he replaced Whitey, Charlie, Sister Hazel, and Ray; he was all of them, rolled into one.

#

In the autumn, I joined Ra at Anderson University. It was a challenge working full time and attending college at night, but it was fun. Dad stopped by one evening after learning that I'd enrolled. He said he was proud of me for trying to better myself and offered to take over the charges and pay my way. I shared with him the actual reason I rejected going to art school in

Chicago; I told him I'd have wasted his money on booze and drugs. I hugged him and thanked him for his offer but declined to accept it as I didn't know if I could keep up the schedule.

A few weeks later, Dad called for me to join him in picking up some material from a local wood mill. When we arrived, the dockhand filled Dad's truck with hundreds of linear feet of custom poplar trim.

I asked Dad what he would do with the woodwork and he said, "It's for your house. I want to help you get it done if I can. I've got you a powered miter saw too; we should be able to make quick work of it."

That's the way he'd always been if given the opportunity. Even when we didn't get along, I'd find tools on my art table; wood chisels, carving knives, expensive pencils, drawing pads, and paintbrushes mysteriously appeared overnight. Over the years, I'd witnessed him pay for his employee's weddings, education, bail, and car payments. If he was at his financial ends, he'd dedicate his free time to the unfortunate. He was a rare soul, and I deeply regretted I'd ever gotten sideways with him. I wished I hadn't been such a lousy person and wasted so many moments with him.

#

In the spring of 1996, Dad's MRI revealed recent tumor growth. To fight it, he chose experimental oral chemotherapy, and it wrecked him. He lost his hair again and couldn't eat. His bodyweight dropped to 136 pounds, and his appearance reminded me of Unck's old friends Jess and Earl.

June was unbearable. Grief and concern shattered Mom. She'd gained weight and her hair was brittle—thinning at its ends—but worse than that, her eyes were blank, revealing the hollowness behind them. She looked like the mother I had in Martinsville, disconnected and broken, but without Dad to help her. She knew what was coming. We all knew what was coming.

Dad's body was failing him. The tumor affected his left side. There was the slightest droop to the corner of his mouth. If the cancer wasn't clenching his hand or drawing it to his sternum, it seemed to tie it to a weight, anchored below his hip, dragging his shoulder with it. He limped and was unsteady. His thoughts were clouded, and he was having episodes of dementia. It was bad enough to see him physically withering, but to witness him panic-stricken, lost in his mind, was brutal. The most powerful entity I'd ever known was faltering, and it was crushing.

#

Mom needed time away from the misery, so on weekends, she ran errands while I visited with Dad. On a Saturday in late September, I sat with him in the living room. In the opposite corner, I turned the TV to a wildlife documentary—the commentator's voice was soothing as he noted the intricacies of life and death in the natural world. Dad seemed to have a good day, although he looked tired. He didn't complain of any pain and was quiet, sitting in his usual contemplative position, with his chin resting on his chest and his hands interlaced on his belly.

When he spoke and said, "It makes sense," I didn't hear him clearly.

"What's that, Pop?"

He responded, "It makes sense."

I expected something simple from him, or maybe he was encountering a bout of dementia that I could steer back to the sunlit room's peacefulness.

I asked, "What makes sense?"

After the slightest pause, he responded, "The dream."

"What dream, Pop?"

"The dream I had about you and Lamech."

"What do you mean, Pop—the old dream?"

He looked at me and said, "I've been thinking about it all morning. Out of all of my children, only you and Lamech remain. You're the last two of my children. I don't know why all of this happened, but it's real. I knew it was important back then, and I've prayed about it all these years. Your names are important. You're the two boys that God revealed to me, and you're the only children I have left. It makes sense. I don't know how, and I don't know why I had that dream, but it finally makes sense."

His clarity struck me as much as his assessment. I hadn't thought of the dream for a long time. It twisted me so profoundly as a boy, I had to leave it there. I accepted it as Dad did; everything about it felt awful. It left me with two undecipherable points; why did two boys appear in the middle of horror, and why did they have unusually specific names? Why the foretelling, and why the names? I could see his correlation; here we were, Dad, Lamech, and Amalek, in the fog of atrocity. Five of his children went to miserable deaths, but the two from a dream remained. Why the names? Were they for Dad or Lamech and me? Amalek—I found it difficult to describe myself as warlike or living in a valley. I'd rolled that title over in my mind so often that I'd rejected it and didn't want any association with it. I could try to ignore it, but as Dad said, I couldn't deny how precise his vision turned out to be.

#

In October, Dad's MRI revealed a complete return of the tumor, and he underwent his second surgery on November 19. He recovered well and came home feeling positive and prepared to continue his fight.

#

On Thanksgiving, November 28, 1996, Ra and I had dinner with her parents and planned on visiting Mom and Dad later that day. On arriving at Lone Oak, we found a note taped to the front storm door, "Took Dad to IU, Mom." I knew the situation was dire; if it were minor, she would have taken him to Riverview. We bundled Morgan back into the car and drove to Indianapolis. After making our way to IU, we went to the reception desk and asked for information. To our confusion, they had no record of admitting anyone with the name of Gadd. We figured Mom must have gone to Riverview and we hurried to Noblesville.

When I passed through the emergency room doors, I could hear Dad screaming. I rushed into his cubicle, where Mom was trying to talk peace into him and hold him in his bed. Lost in misery and agony, he writhed and cried about being on fire. Mom quickly explained that Dad awakened in pain earlier in the afternoon and thought someone had shot him in the head. He was inconsolable, and his condition worsened. She knew to take him to IU but couldn't manage him and drive, so she diverted to Riverview. She was desperate and complained that the ER staff refused to give him any morphine because they couldn't confirm the source of Dad's torment. Hours later, they contacted IU, who recommended his transfer. He was still wailing when they loaded him in the ambulance.

At IU, they scanned his body for blood clots and ran him through the CT machine again but found no cause for his pain. Dad was fitful and out of his mind. Throughout the night, Mom, Ra, and I took turns tending to Dad and Morgan. He was in and out of consciousness, screaming and whimpering, clawing at his head.

With the morning shift change, they noticed his elevated white cell count and administered a spinal tap. Within minutes, a doctor entered the waiting room and told us that Dad's spinal fluid was cloudy instead of clear and that it was most likely meningitis.

With this information, they sedated Dad, placed him on life support, and mounted a campaign to fight the infection.

#

The next three weeks were brutal. Mom checked into a nearby hotel to be as close to Dad as she could. I went to work each morning, to IU each evening, and returned home each night to sleep and shower. On a few nights, I attended my classes at Anderson University, but it was pointless. I couldn't focus; it all paled compared to what was happening to Dad.

The interactions with family, acquaintances, and church folk were stressful; everyone wanted Dad to survive as much as anyone else did. Their challenges with fear and grief rolled over into petty disagreements and tiffs with one another. It was physically and emotionally draining to explain Dad's condition to each visitor. I appreciated their love for him, hell, we all loved him! He was a magnificent soul, and we pined to have him back, whole as he'd always been. We were all grasping at the same rope, but it was slick with water and mire, and it was anchored somewhere that none of us could ever go to release it.

It wore on us, and we said things we didn't mean or want to be real. All you could do was cry at the tubes in Dad's mouth and arms and plead with him to wake up, but you knew he couldn't and most likely wouldn't. We recognized we were helpless. You could press your spirit at it, pray until you couldn't any longer, and appeal to the stars for a turnaround, but in the pit of your stomach, you understood you were up against something that had a momentum of its own and you couldn't stop it. You'd find yourself whispering to Dad, wanting to believe those ideas that the unconscious can hear you. You'd recount past events and speak of happenings in the lives of those around him, and make sure you mentioned everyone that was there praying for him, hoping some little word might resonate and stir him to health. Still, the only responses were the rhythmic sounds of his respirator against his heart monitor.

#

On Monday, December 17, 1996, Mom called me at work. She was crying and said she couldn't get hold of Lamech. She admitted that Dad wasn't going to come back, and she knew he wouldn't want to exist this way; he'd written a living will that refused extraordinary measures to keep him alive. When she asked what I thought, I felt like a boy again, holding a wounded dove, staring into its coal-colored eyes. I realized what she was asking, and it broke my heart. I never expected to be in a position to put my father down. Being the youngest child, I didn't feel I had any stake in the decision until I remembered there wasn't anyone around anymore but me.

She asked again what I thought, and I said, "Let's let him go, Momma. I'll be there in a minute."

Later that day, when they removed Dad from life support and gave him a little morphine, his countenance calmed, and he was peaceful. We transferred him to Riverview to be closer to home and set up a watch.

On December 19, I'd come home to shower when Mom called and said I needed to return as Dad's heart rate had declined.

We watched him throughout the afternoon. He was quiet and comfortable, breathing shallowly with interminable pauses between respirations. The few remaining members and friends of the Gadd clan whispered wishes and farewells to Dad. As with my brothers and sisters, each pause between breaths was a hurtful misery bound with a hope that pined for it to be the last.

Dad's final breath eventually came and went out of him, and a few moments later, his spirit left us. We held his hands, touched his forehead, and felt the coldness settle.

He'd lived almost three months past his fifty-seventh birthday. It was hurtful to realize he'd not only borne the deaths of his children, but also physically experienced their every misery.

#

Dad's funeral, like Joe's three years previously, was a few days before Christmas. Our figurehead was gone, and so was our momentum. Mom turned over the duties of planning his memorial to me. We hosted the service for Dad at a mortuary in Anderson, where I made sure to meet everyone at the door and accepted their condolences.

We carried his body to Martinsville and interred him next to Garnna, Shelam, and Joe. His remains rested not only with his departed children but also the members of the community that raised him. If those old souls could have voiced their opinions, I'm sure they would honor him. Like a stanza from one of Dad's favorite poems, his head was bloody but unbowed.

CHAPTER 9

The Dark
1997 (26 Years Old)

AFTER DAD'S FUNERAL, the light went out inside me, and I didn't care to see anything anymore. I returned to work and dropped out of school. I worked on the house every evening, but it was half-hearted. I quit playing music and drawing. Sleeping through the night was difficult. I had recurring dreams of murdering Dad in the shed behind the garage on Lone Oak Road. I'm not sure how many nights I put a gun to his head, pulled the trigger, and tried to keep his brains from pouring out of the holes in his skull.

I didn't notice winter transitioning to spring. Memorial Day came, and we visited Dad's gravesite. His gray granite stone next to Joe's, Shelam's, and Garnna's matched my heart.

I didn't concern myself with anybody around me or think to assess how Dad's death affected them until Mom asked Lamech, Ra, and me to join her for family therapy sessions. We all went a few times, but it seemed fruitless. I could see the counselor struggling to unpack the damage we all contained. I felt sorry for her; she did her best, but she was out of her depth. I didn't want to be a hurdle for anyone and preferred not to talk about my story, so I quit going.

#

Before Dad died, they tested Lamech for the Gadds' genetic anomaly; the outcome was negative, so he'd dodged the bullet. I put the query off, out of financial obligations and fear. After Dad died, Mom and Ra pressed me to discover what might or might not be within me. I met with Dad's doctor and she explained the process. I had my blood drawn and in a few weeks, I received the results. I opened the envelope and unfolded the letter. A few paragraphs reiterated my desire for the test, described the test performed, and illuminated the lack of a mutation at gene P53. I wasn't a carrier and had no mutation to pass to any offspring. I didn't know how to accept this information. I wasn't excited or relieved. I thought I'd experience euphoria over not having the threat on my shoulders anymore, but I felt something foreign, and I couldn't clearly explain to Ra or anyone what it was.

#

Some mornings, on the way to work, I'd notice Dad passing me in his station wagon. A few times, I saw him in line ahead of me at the grocery store, slipping through the crowd, just out of reach.

I operated on autopilot, not knowing how or when I arrived at work or made it home. I started drinking as I did in high school, except I had access to a larger volume and didn't

THE BIRD'S ROAD   219

have to hide it. Ra worked nights at Bonge's Tavern and after I tucked Morgan into bed, I'd open a bottle of liquor and finish it just short of falling asleep, not caring if I'd wake up or not.

I was sensible enough to know I had a problem but didn't understand how far away I was from the shore. I couldn't wipe the things I'd seen from my eyes, and they haunted me while I was awake, through the night, and even while out of my mind.

When the autumn came, I felt the first splintering fissures of collapse. Like the weight of water undermining a foundation, every little and enormous thing that was ever hurtful, the events I'd never considered because I never knew how, and all the injuries I'd shunted into a reservoir of forgetfulness, compounded under pressure and bored their way through.

I thought since these things were in my past and there was no future of misery or death, there was some divide or potential insulation between them and me and then and now. I believed I could take the time to open some of these memories and try to make friends with them.

Unfortunately, I didn't know that I didn't have the tools, emotional maturity, or fortitude to handle the smallest event. Also, I didn't realize that unbolting the lock for one memory permitted all of them to cascade from their chamber. Initially, they dazzled me, as they shined with love, but soon I wanted to put my eyes out. They roared, screamed, and pounded down on me like a torrent from a failed dam, and I could neither swim nor find the surface. In the murkiness and turbulence, I realized something was tied to my neck, holding me under, and I couldn't free myself from it. That chain was the prognosis of my genetic testing. At first, it offered a long existence without the worries and dread I'd lived with for thirteen years. Now, it was a realization that I'd wasted my life, was unprepared for any good fortune, and wasn't of the same fiber as those who were gone. I was underwater. I blew out the air I had remaining in my lungs and the water came pouring in.

#

On a day in October, I visited our family physician for an infected cut across my knuckles. He'd cared for Joe, Danny, and Dad and was acquainted with our family's struggles.

As he scrubbed my hand, he pointedly asked me, "Sharek, do you ever feel like going away on a long drive without telling anyone or ever wonder what it might be like if you weren't here anymore?"

"Yeah, I think about that. Mostly, I want it all to go away; I don't want to have ever been around."

When he laid the nonstick pad on my hand and wrapped it with tape, he asked, "Whenever you feel that way again, and you've got the keys in your hand, would you call me?" He pulled a page from the notebook he kept in his lab coat, wrote a number on it, and said, "Any time, day or night, call me—no questions asked—and I'll give you a hand."

I flashed back to a rain-drenched fishing trip with Charlie and remembered Ray's firm hand on my shoulder. I looked at the doc and said, "I'll try."

#

When numbers and letters on pages started rearranging themselves, words seemed misspelled, and equations I'd used for years stopped making sense, I knew something was wrong. For several days, I sat at my drafting table and stared blankly at work piling up. I realized there was nothing I could do. I couldn't function anymore.

A few days passed, and I made the call to Dad's doctor. He met me at Riverview Hospital, set me up in a room, and gave me Demerol. The next morning, he transferred me to a stress center in Indianapolis. I was there for two weeks, sitting in group discussions and one-on-one sessions with the host physician. I listened to the group leader trying to get anybody to talk. She gave out sheets of printer paper and asked everyone to draw pictures of their feelings. She experimented with several methods, most likely well researched and approved, but her young age and lack of experience were detrimental. She even wrote me a prescription for antidepressants, but I didn't believe medication could fix me.

They discharged me on October 30, and I reported to work on Halloween. As soon as I arrived, the company president called me into his office and terminated me for weak performance and poor attendance. He suggested it might do me some good to find Jesus. I nodded, exited his office, gathered my drawing tools from my desk, and left the building.

#

I was out of work and not inclined to find more. I'd never learned to invest in planning a future, not even a few months in advance. I estimated I could cover our bills for a limited time by selling my guitars and amplifiers. I took most of my gear to IRC Music on 82nd Street in Castleton, where they gave me bottom dollar. It pinched a little to turn it all over, but I figured I didn't need it anymore. From there, I went across the road to pay off a loan and noticed a military recruiting station.

#

The previous summer, I'd taken up reading war stories and explored the exploits of Rangers, Green Berets, and Navy SEALS. Their history and challenges sparked something inside me. Everything about it felt similar to what I missed; the qualities of brotherhood, danger, extreme situations, and facing an enemy on a battlefield sang like a siren to my soul. Shortly after Dad died, I connected with Dad's brother, Uncle Bill, and we talked each week. During World War II, he was a Naval Scout/Raider. He was stationed in the Pacific, covertly occupying islands under Japanese control. After the war, he enlisted in the Army. On March 23, 1951, he received a battlefield commission on the first of two airborne insertions during the Korean War.

#

When the town of Lapel cut power to the house, I took my last Gibson Les Paul to IRC and let it go for five hundred dollars. On the way home, I drove by the military recruiting station. I'd been mulling over enlisting and, frankly, it was the only prospect of earning a wage that appealed to me. I stepped inside to look around. Thinking about Uncle Bill, I went to talk to the Navy recruiter. He laid out a marvelous story, but being confined to a ship for six months out of a year sounded miserable. The Marine recruiter was at an appointment. I wasn't interested in reaching for the sky, so I walked past the Air Force office and knocked on the Army recruiter's door. Up front, he was honest and said he didn't want to discuss anything until I completed a physical and the Armed Services Vocational Aptitude Battery.

I drove back home and stopped by the town office to pay off our utility bill. The following day, I called Uncle Bill and shared my thoughts about joining the Army. I told him I didn't feel fit to live. He knew where I'd been since losing Dad and spoke truth to me.

He said, "Do what you feel like doing. The Army isn't a bad decision; you can get sorted out there, and they'll take care of your family. If that's what you want to do, don't worry about anything else. Do what it takes to stay alive."

I told Ra about the possibility of joining the Army but, justifiably, she wasn't on board. A few days later, the recruiter drove me to Indianapolis Military Entrance Processing Station, where I passed my physical and scored high on the ASVAB. After another visit to the recruitment office, I contracted for a guaranteed station with the 101st Airborne at Fort Campbell, Kentucky. I signed on with a $12,000 bonus and the promise of a paycheck hitting Ra's bank account within a couple of weeks of in-processing. I figured that would hold me as close to home as possible and permit us to keep our house in Lapel.

I didn't tell Ra until after I enlisted. The following days were heartbreaking, but I failed to see any other option. I was splintered, and the world around me was dark except that little light of potential challenge the military offered. I broke her heart and Morgan's; we'd never spent more than a few nights away from each other. I knew I'd return to them, but I had no way to convince Ra. She asked me to pack all my things and store them in the attic in case anything foul happened. As a testament to her exceptional qualities, even though she believed I was ripping everything apart, she supported me.

#

In the early morning hours on January 26, 1998, I woke, dressed, and picked up the pack of clothes my recruiter told me to bring. I walked the few steps to Morgan's room and kissed her forehead as she slept. Ra followed me downstairs to the living room, and we embraced. When I heard a vehicle rolling into our gravel driveway, I kissed Ra and backed out the front door, searing into my brain the vision of leaving her standing on a cold hardwood floor.

My recruiter drove me to MEPS. After swearing my oath, I departed in a limousine with a few other recruits. On arrival at the bus station, we shook hands and went our separate ways. A few were heading to Naval Station Great Lakes, and some were on their way to the East Coast to become Marines. I was traveling to Fort Knox for Basic and Advanced Individual Training.

#

I boarded a Greyhound bus that took what seemed like an eternity to transport me and my small backpack to central Kentucky. Throughout the day, the rolling carcass rumbled to stop at its prepositioned hubs and disgorged the other travelers. Now, but for the driver, I was unaccompanied.

As the miles accumulated on the odometer, my old life slipped away. Leaving it hurt, but then again, so did staying. Back there was a world full of memories that I couldn't think about anymore; when I did, they crippled me.

I didn't want to die, necessarily, but I didn't want to live with all the awful things I'd witnessed and done. As long as I could remember, my life always felt one way—some other course but mine. I'd taken it all and rolled with it, but in the process, I got messed up and failed to figure a direction. I had a core group of loving and helpful people beside me, but I couldn't shake the feeling of being alone and expired. They desired to save me, but I refused to let them cover themselves in my grime. Anyway, how could they know how to help me? I reckoned you could love someone into a better state of mind about as well as you could love the dying away from death. I didn't want to be anybody's burden, and I didn't want any pity.

My brokenness angered me. My weakness disgusted me. I was done being in that shark cage from my childhood dreams.

I refused to fear the leviathans on the other side of the bars. I gave up worrying about not being tethered to the surface. It seemed since the time I was born, my destiny wasn't to breathe a normal person's air, and now I didn't care. If it wanted me to swim in the deep, I would, and while down there, I'd hunt those monsters.

I needed another world, one that offered something similar to the severity of the old one. I wasn't afraid of dying; I'd bathed in that emotional response since I was nine years old. I understood I wouldn't succumb to the same fate as my deceased loved ones; that kind of dying didn't want me. Since it was clear my death would play out in some other way, I'd choose its stage. I decided to meet the benefactor of my father's dream on the terms it authored. I'd run counter to how I was raised and be what they named me. I'd press the veil that separates this existence from the next and tempt that faceless void into face-to-face engagement.

#

The bus lumbered to a halt on a small hill next to a battered concrete hut, opened its maw, and spit me from its gullet. I stepped out into the gloom of a growing storm. The transport pulled away as a damp wind picked up red dust from the ground and flicked it against me.

Lightning flashed in the distance, silhouetting the unfamiliar horizon in crimson and gold. Thunder rumbled and mingled with the unmistakable "boom" and "krump" of artillery rising and falling in faraway fields.

I stood, inhaling the cordite, ozone, and rain in the hollow of night. The atmosphere charged me, causing the hair on my neck to stand on end.

I'd received no instructions on what to do after arriving. I figured I'd now be face to face with a drill instructor, but the hilltop was utterly vacant of life. With no one to greet me, the thought of slipping away flashed through my mind. I could escape from this plan—evade into the forest, and no one would observe my parting—but I had no place to go. I'd committed myself to this path and left my home and all it had to offer. I wasn't prepared for any other option.

I looked at my surroundings more closely. Under the steel canopy over the entrance to the hut—illuminated by a dim lamp—was a hinged metal box stenciled with faded yellow paint, "Unaccompanied Arrivals." I walked to it and raised the cover, revealing a scarred telephone from a previous war. The receiver wore varied shades of olive, and below its base was a single illuminated red button.

This moment was final; the terminal seconds it would take my finger to touch the blood-colored button would be my last as the person I was. The device was bitter against my ear. My chest expanded as I formulated words for the being on the other end of the line. I exhaled old worries as my heart rushed and resonated in my ears. I looked into the imminent roar, drew one last breath, and depressed the flaming contact that would announce my arrival.

Another flash in the blackness, another rumble, more thunder.

ADDENDUM

2016 (45 Years Old)

I DROVE WEST to Harbor Manor through the remnants of an August rain. The sky broke in bands of charcoal to expose the golden light of a setting sun. The road curved through a creek bottom where deer grazed in a fallow field with a blanket of dew suspended above their red backs.

Harbor Manor is where Mom lay in hospice while calling for her life to be over. I kept the night watch as I was nearest the rest home and couldn't sleep knowing she was alone.

A misplaced step led her there; several years earlier, she'd fallen and broken her hip. A brace of clumsy surgeons further damaged her condition until, by chance, after ten surgeries, bacteria took hold of her and refused to let go. She'd entered the hospital the previous Memorial Day and rejected plans to amputate her leg. She accepted a method of intravenous treatment and steeled herself against everyone's emotions by stating that she didn't want to pass, but if she did, it was God's will. Her granddaughters protested, and her friends questioned her mental stability, but she remained immovable. She was exhausted and critically depressed. She asked for my support. I challenged her by questioning her willingness to die from an infection; I hoped that the thoughts of a protracted and painful death might shake her from her decision. I knew she'd thought through the scenario—she'd been around this level of desperation most of her life—and I expected her confident response. She wasn't going to live as an amputee.

#

During the month of June, her condition rose and sank on swells of septicemia. Her white blood cell count was more than double a human's top limit, and the open wound in her leg would not heal. She crossed the event horizon and moved toward the singularity of death.

#

On a sultry morning in July, her doctor called me to her bedside to sign a Do Not Resuscitate Declaration. Ra met me in the foyer outside Mom's room. We talked with the physician and the convalescence practitioners. They convinced us—by Mom's condition—that she had few days left.

While the staff went to prepare the documents, Ra and I entered Mom's room. Though it was bright and clean, the suite trapped the odor of infection. Through the venetian blinds on the window, the sun lay across her face. She was as beautiful as she'd always been. With my thumb, I traced the structure of her brow and temples that so closely matched her mother's. Mom hadn't colored her hair in months, and it was taking on a silvery luster. She slowly opened her once brilliant blue eyes—they'd been gray and lackluster for several weeks—and tried to focus on mine. The crow's-feet at the corners of her eyes expanded as she recognized me.

As she trapped my gaze, a flickering slideshow featuring her ran through my mind; I experienced a trillion moments we'd shared. Her wrinkles seemed to fade, and her eyes lost the fog of death. I saw her when she was sixty and I was thirty—a year older than Carrie, Danny, or Joe ever became. She was fifty-five and Dad was gone. She was fifty-one and we were at the hospital as Danny took his last breath. She was forty-nine and Joe was struggling to stay alive. She was forty-seven and petting Carrie's lifeless hand. She was forty-two, in the backyard, posing for photos on her twenty-fifth wedding anniversary. She was thirty and cradling me in a cold cabin, looking down on my dying sister. She was twenty-eight and running out of a laundromat with Shelam in her arms. She was nineteen, clutching Dad, as she wept beside Garnna's grave in Martinsville. She was sixteen, holding Dad's hand on her wedding day. She was six, drinking Coke from a bottle as she leaned against the fender of her brother's car. She was an infant, searching her mother's eyes, the same way I was trying to find purchase in hers.

As she had my entire life, she said, "Hey, Shrimp."

"Hey, Momma."

She asked, "What's going on—why's the doctor still here?"

"I gotta talk to you about something."

"Why's the doctor still here?"

"That's what I've got to talk to you about."

She'd seen her doctor earlier that morning and saw him again as Ra and I entered the room. Shockingly, her moments of clarity came abruptly and powerfully. She could exist for several days with minimal function, seemingly unconscious, but then surprise everyone with a rally of health that was odd and disturbing.

She asked, and I couldn't do anything but tell her. Again, I felt the cold that comes over one's heart when you have to push away emotion—much like an accomplished surgeon dismisses distraction while piercing flesh with a scalpel—accepting the responsibility for the death of life in your hands.

I was a boy again, trying to wipe beads of crimson from the feathers of a mourning dove I'd shot.

I remembered the moment, twenty years previously, when Mom and I determined to remove Dad from life support.

My pause was lengthy, and she asked again, "What's going on?"

She instantly knew and shrank into tears as I said, "Momma, we're at the end, and the doctors can't do any more for you." I felt the dove struggle in my hand.

She asked, "Can I change my mind?"

"Momma, it's too late, you'd never survive the operation."

With earnestness, as if it were an original idea, she pleaded, "Tell 'em to take my leg!"

"It's too late."

She whimpered, "I want to live!"

"I know you do, Momma."

"But I want to live!"

"I know, Momma."

Agonizingly, she wept until her eyes dried. Then she furrowed her brow and asked, "Why am I here?"

Again, as I had at least twice a week since she'd been in this state, I recounted the previous months and our conversations. I told her about all of her loved ones who had visited her. I described her last surgery, the chronology of the events that led to her confinement at Harbor Manor, the infection that now racked her body, the terminal direction of her affairs, and her decision to have no further medical interventions.

My response seemed to settle her, but I wondered if she was asking the larger question. Why was she here? It was pointless to ask why this road was ending where it was. I traced the veins on Mom's needle-bruised hands and felt cold hate for our situation. I saw no reason in the dying. Senseless deaths laid out behind us like fresh laundry, blown from the line, lying in the mud. All the bright and all the shine extinguished with fewer of us each season to remember the glow. I reckon it's just what our lot meant for us to do: watch each other waste away until we're nothing but husks—our teeth grinding in dry mouths with wet cheeks, pleading for the other not to suffer. It wore and misshaped us like old whetstones, but what did we sharpen? What comes from sick and stricken children or a mother and a father burying all their babies? What comes of a boy watching them all die? I can tell you, not a damn thing. Not one goddamn thing. What's the gold to pan from all of this? It's a pan full of grave dirt saturated with tears, rolled around in an icy stream of grief, and sifted for a minuscule glimmer that might feed your empty heart, but there's never anything there.

We never fell apart. We transcended exhibiting emotions. We mastered not hoping for much. We held low expectations. We proficiently kept a distance from others. We versed ourselves in funerals. We refused to let paltry things get to us. We excelled at not talking. We maintained a proper appearance and an ability to go through the motions of living. All the while, we died inside.

Mom's multiyear disability tired her, but that wasn't the only weariness within her. That's what no one seemed to realize, or at least they failed to talk about it. I saw it, but I didn't know how to shoulder it. I'd experienced that infrasound groan that emanated from her since I was a baby. I didn't need to see it; I felt it. It's how I'd always known her. Mothers sing to their babies. I knew her song.

Again, she broke into sobs. With no idea what to say, I asked her to talk.

She raised her other hand and wept, "I'm a chicken! I've come all this way, and at the end, I break—I'm a chicken!"

"Mom, you're not a chicken, you're the most powerful person I've known."

"No, I'm not—I'm a chicken!"

The physician knocked on the door and entered the room. With compassion, he explained the situation to Mom and asked her if she understood. She wiped her eyes and nose with a balled-up tissue and confirmed that she did. He passed us the DNR printed in black with the areas we needed to sign highlighted in yellow. I read its verbiage and signed it, and Mom applied her signature. I handed it to the doctor, he departed, and we were quiet.

#

Days wore on, and the medical staff tried to manage her suffering, but it frustrated them. They administered a staggering quantity of opiates and antianxiety medication, but she remained restless and writhed in agony.

#

One morning, hours before dawn, I realized why she consistently cried out in fits of torment, "It hurts so bad!" We were fighting the wrong pain.

After the nurses prepared her for the night, I turned out the lights, moved my chair against her bedside, and settled for my shift. Fitfully, she slept a few hours. I watched the stars rise above the trees outside her window. She writhed from sleep with a moan and rolled her head back and forth across her pillow.

"What's wrong, Momma?" I asked.

"It hurts so bad."

"Do you want the nurse?"

"No …," she groaned. The dim light coming through the window illuminated tears running from the corners of her eyes.

I pulled a tissue from the nightstand for her, held her hand, and asked, "Momma, what hurts?"

She hesitated, with her eyes seeming to bore holes through the ceiling. Then she groaned and said, "All of it."

"All of what?"

She rolled her head to face me, her eyes red and wet, and whispered, "I'm so sorry."

"Sorry for what, Momma?"

"I'm sorry you had to grow up the way you did … I'm sorry I wasn't there for you."

I felt a new fissure form across my heart. "Momma, I'm okay … you and Pop couldn't do anything about that—I understood it back then."

"But it hurts me that you were so alone …"

"It's okay, Momma; I've felt no kind of bad about you and Dad not being around—there's no way you could have—I knew where you needed to be … I knew it way back then."

She whispered, "… I'm so sorry."

"Let that go right now—that's not anything I've ever held."

She wiped her raw eyes, looked above my head as if she were searching for a face in a crowd, and whispered through her trembling lips, "It all hurts so bad …"

She broke into sobs, "… Garnna was gone so quick—Shelam was so beautiful—I couldn't do anything to save her …"

Like a smack to the face, I acutely realized the source of her untreatable pain. The grief and sorrow that poured out of her went through me like a spear. I held my words and let her unravel.

"... Joe didn't deserve that—he was so strong." She pressed her forearm across her eyes as if to remove the vision. She shook with convulsions of agony, her mouth agape, groaning and weeping.

"... and Danny ... they didn't deserve that!"

"... oh God ... it hurts so bad!"

"... and Carrie ... Carrie—it was so cruel."

"She was my best friend ... she was so wonderful." She forced herself to be calm and gouged at her eyes with a collection of tissues. Again, she searched the space behind me. She finally focused on me, and her lips trembled as she spoke, "I miss her so bad."

"I do too, Momma."

"Sharek, I'm so sorry."

"Me too, Momma."

Her eyes—locked on mine—flowed again. Her heartbreaking confession continued, "... she was so wonderful—I miss her so bad ..."

"... and I couldn't do anything to save her."

"I died when Carrie died."

"Dad broke, and we couldn't do anything for each other."

"It all hurts so bad ..." She rocked her head from side to side with her eyes closed.

"It all hurts so bad ..."

"It all hurts so bad."

Broken, I said, "It was all very cruel, Momma."

"Yes, it was, Sharek—yes, it was." Her wave of emotion subsided, and she dabbed her eyes, saying, "Dad would be so proud of you ... He loved you so much."

"I miss him, Momma."

"I know you do." She was quiet, looking through me as if I weren't there, and she was in a different place. I saw what she was seeing: their faces, both laughing and in repose. I felt all the horrible loss. I remembered the ends they all met and the ultimate moments when their breath failed to return. I considered the words I wished I'd said and phrases I wanted to hear from them before they slipped away. I felt as if a window and shutters were closing to hide the starlight. "Momma … I'll miss you."

Knowing what I was thinking, she responded, "I'll miss you, Shrimp."

#

Her sorrow, so close to the surface, shouldn't have surprised me. I'd gotten used to not fully feeling mine, and I thought she had too. It made sense at this point. She knew she was dying.

Now, standing at the edge of darkness, she turned to look at where she'd been and completely embraced all she had to hold. She let the memories in.

#

When she was physically healthy, she never complained. In front of most everyone, she kept a beaming smile and cheerful disposition. The more tribulation assailed her, the more she proclaimed her faith and God's ability to heal her wounds. She volunteered for church activities and donated her time to compassionate programs or others struggling with life.

She opened her home to acquaintances and strangers, and they flocked to her. I'm not sure if they wanted to help her or not. Maybe they had a fascination, like someone who visits a roadside attraction to see something from the dark of a jungle. Some people kneeled at her feet, hoping to find aid for their damage.

Everyone plied their ability at compassion by recalling memories of Joe or Dad. It was the easiest way to show they cared, but holding up a fragment of what once was is like knocking at the door of sorrow without the intention of ever entering the room. Some could lay out their troubles with hers, but they splashed along the shore of a great depth.

If you didn't know her past, you'd never surmise she'd experienced so many tragic events. If you were familiar with her history, it wasn't something easily placed on the table for conversation. If you witnessed what she'd gone through, you'd not likely wade in her waters.

She swam in a kind of ocean that seemed to have no shore. She drifted out in the bottomless, dark, and uncharted region where horrific objects lay anchored below the surface. Over the years, I'd tried to make my way to her, but I found myself further away with each stroke as if there were a current that worked against us. There was a point where we almost reached one another, but there were overwhelming beasts out there, and I was too young and inexperienced to wrestle them. By the time I was capable, she was too far away for me to grasp.

You'd think we survivors, Mom, Lamech, and me—having endured what we had—would be closer to one another and have long intimate talks about the things that hurt us and spend every available moment together. We talked, but it was always fragmented. Our gatherings were like trying to repair a torn picture; the fuzzy and twisted edges never align the right way, and the essential shapes are missing.

So much transpired over such an interminable period, it felt pointless and burdensome to dig through what was. Anyway, we knew what happened, and we knew what it did to us. That was unquestionable. Mostly, I think being near each other made it all real again. We were each a testament of what bloodied us and being face to face brought out the feelings of being back in some emergency room, hospital cafeteria, mortuary, or graveside. Frankly, that's where we'd spent our most emotionally significant periods. Having lived with one another at that pinnacle of severity made every other moment that much less fulfilling.

I never felt I was what she needed. I believe she cared for me and most likely loved me, but as magnets opposed, we remained out of reach. I knew I couldn't save her.

Now, she wasn't in the ocean; she was the ocean.

Again, waiting beside the dying, I wonder what's on the other side. I chance to think it could be like waking in Mamaw's house with my forehead under Unck's gentle hand. From there, it's just a quick walk through the dark to the kitchen's warm glow. Perhaps all of them are there. Danny and Joe, wet with snow from delivering newspapers. Carrie, with Mamaw, at the stove making cocoa. Dad is there, bouncing Shelam on his lap. Maybe Mom's walking up to the porch right now, with Garnna bundled in her arms. I feel a shoulder against mine as Lamech joins me, and we're as close as veterans can be. No one is marked, and there is no memory or foresight of what was or would be.

Perhaps it's just a fade into an endless dark, until we rise anew as undulating grasses on a field, or as trees, waving in the sky. If fortunate, maybe something larger takes us, and again, we find our way to a womb and wake as some other life.

Though I like to imagine being with all of them again, after the dark, I think what we know of nature is the reality; it's the only ending for us, that is a beautiful truth.

Ultimately, I think it's akin to what Dad told me on a cool September morning as, hand in hand, he led me to look into the sky and see the Bird's Road. I believe he shared the foundational truth that day, but he was vague on the critical point: we are already there, suffused into that velvety field of stars along the raised arm of Orion. Everyone that was is still here now, in this present moment; we comprise them, both genetically and in our thoughts and actions. The people and experiences that shaped them affect us, and the ripple continues across the water to a shore we'll never see.

Looking to where I came from and the distance between then and now is like observing a trail of stepping stones through a twisting stream; each foothold is a point in time where some character imparted a lesson to me, knowingly or not. That education—the human connection—is the only secret to living, and it's waiting there for everyone, in plain sight.

I let almost fifty years go by without realizing what Pop always tried to get me to understand. Maybe if things hadn't gone in the direction they did, I wouldn't have gotten so rounded off and could have developed the character a common way of living affords, along with some sensibility in my conclusions. Perhaps the realization that my life matters would have come to me sooner, and I'd have stopped battering my wounds and cutting away the parts of me that hurt.

Weighing these thoughts against where I've walked—if there's anything that tips the balance and needs sharing with everyone, it's these points. Recognize that you are the most valuable resource you possess, and your engagement with other people matters. You have the ability to endure and overcome more than you could ever imagine. Every day is worth experiencing, and you've earned knowledge that can restore a damaged person. Be the good that someone gave to you, and if you've never known such compassion, be the kind of human that you needed in your darkest hour.

As my Pop would say, "You'll be bettered by it."

GRAND PATRONS

Scott Bardash
Mitch Davis
Mark T. Duffin
Lorelei Farlow
Ryan and Shannon Funke
Morgan Gadd
RaAnn Gadd
Andy Keffaber
Alysha Renee Klees
Donald and Katherine Kroger
Alan T. Rose Jr
Jeri Rusk
Brian Toombs
Joel and Kiersten Tragesser
Christopher Wirthwein
Dawn Zapinski

INKSHARES

INKSHARES is a reader-driven publisher and producer based in Oakland, California. Our books are selected not by a group of editors, but by readers worldwide.

While we've published books by established writers like *Big Fish* author Daniel Wallace and *Star Wars: Rogue One* scribe Gary Whitta, our aim remains surfacing and developing the new author voices of tomorrow.

Previously unknown Inkshares authors have received starred reviews and been featured in the *New York Times*. Their books are on the front tables of Barnes & Noble and hundreds of independents nationwide, and many have been licensed by publishers in other major markets. They are also being adapted by Oscar-winning screenwriters at the biggest studios and networks.

Interested in making your own story a reality? Visit Inkshares.com to start your own project or find other great books.